My Personal In

Name ....

Phone ....

Address

....

....

My Emergency contacts

1 ....

....

2 ....

....

3 ....

....

Weekly Diabetes Record

Name: _____

Date:	Breakfast	Snack	Lunch	Snack	Dinner	Snack	Bedtime	Night	Notes
Blood Sugar									
Insulin Dose									
Grams Carb									
Activity									

Date:	Breakfast	Snack	Lunch	Snack	Dinner	Snack	Bedtime	Night	Notes
Blood Sugar									
Insulin Dose									
Grams Carb									
Activity									

Date:	Breakfast	Snack	Lunch	Snack	Dinner	Snack	Bedtime	Night	Notes
Blood Sugar									
Insulin Dose									
Grams Carb									
Activity									

Date:	Breakfast	Snack	Lunch	Snack	Dinner	Snack	Bedtime	Night	Notes
Blood Sugar									
Insulin Dose									
Grams Carb									
Activity									

Date:	Breakfast	Snack	Lunch	Snack	Dinner	Snack	Bedtime	Night	Notes
Blood Sugar									
Insulin Dose									
Grams Carb									
Activity									

Date:	Breakfast	Snack	Lunch	Snack	Dinner	Snack	Bedtime	Night	Notes
Blood Sugar									
Insulin Dose									
Grams Carb									
Activity									

Date:	Breakfast	Snack	Lunch	Snack	Dinner	Snack	Bedtime	Night	Notes
Blood Sugar									
Insulin Dose									
Grams Carb									
Activity									

Weekly Diabetes Record

Name:

Date:	Breakfast	Snack	Lunch	Snack	Dinner	Snack	Bedtime	Night	Notes
Blood Sugar									
Insulin Dose									
Grams Carb									
Activity									

Date:	Breakfast	Snack	Lunch	Snack	Dinner	Snack	Bedtime	Night	Notes
Blood Sugar									
Insulin Dose									
Grams Carb									
Activity									

Date:	Breakfast	Snack	Lunch	Snack	Dinner	Snack	Bedtime	Night	Notes
Blood Sugar									
Insulin Dose									
Grams Carb									
Activity									

Date:	Breakfast	Snack	Lunch	Snack	Dinner	Snack	Bedtime	Night	Notes
Blood Sugar									
Insulin Dose									
Grams Carb									
Activity									

Date:	Breakfast	Snack	Lunch	Snack	Dinner	Snack	Bedtime	Night	Notes
Blood Sugar									
Insulin Dose									
Grams Carb									
Activity									

Date:	Breakfast	Snack	Lunch	Snack	Dinner	Snack	Bedtime	Night	Notes
Blood Sugar									
Insulin Dose									
Grams Carb									
Activity									

Date:	Breakfast	Snack	Lunch	Snack	Dinner	Snack	Bedtime	Night	Notes
Blood Sugar									
Insulin Dose									
Grams Carb									
Activity									

Weekly Diabetes Record

Name: _____

Date:	Breakfast	Snack	Lunch	Snack	Dinner	Snack	Bedtime	Night	Notes
Blood Sugar									
Insulin Dose									
Grams Carb									
Activity									

Date:	Breakfast	Snack	Lunch	Snack	Dinner	Snack	Bedtime	Night	Notes
Blood Sugar									
Insulin Dose									
Grams Carb									
Activity									

Date:	Breakfast	Snack	Lunch	Snack	Dinner	Snack	Bedtime	Night	Notes
Blood Sugar									
Insulin Dose									
Grams Carb									
Activity									

Date:	Breakfast	Snack	Lunch	Snack	Dinner	Snack	Bedtime	Night	Notes
Blood Sugar									
Insulin Dose									
Grams Carb									
Activity									

Date:	Breakfast	Snack	Lunch	Snack	Dinner	Snack	Bedtime	Night	Notes
Blood Sugar									
Insulin Dose									
Grams Carb									
Activity									

Date:	Breakfast	Snack	Lunch	Snack	Dinner	Snack	Bedtime	Night	Notes
Blood Sugar									
Insulin Dose									
Grams Carb									
Activity									

Date:	Breakfast	Snack	Lunch	Snack	Dinner	Snack	Bedtime	Night	Notes
Blood Sugar									
Insulin Dose									
Grams Carb									
Activity									

Weekly Diabetes Record

Name:

Date:	Breakfast	Snack	Lunch	Snack	Dinner	Snack	Bedtime	Night	Notes
Blood Sugar									
Insulin Dose									
Grams Carb									
Activity									

Date:	Breakfast	Snack	Lunch	Snack	Dinner	Snack	Bedtime	Night	Notes
Blood Sugar									
Insulin Dose									
Grams Carb									
Activity									

Date:	Breakfast	Snack	Lunch	Snack	Dinner	Snack	Bedtime	Night	Notes
Blood Sugar									
Insulin Dose									
Grams Carb									
Activity									

Date:	Breakfast	Snack	Lunch	Snack	Dinner	Snack	Bedtime	Night	Notes
Blood Sugar									
Insulin Dose									
Grams Carb									
Activity									

Date:	Breakfast	Snack	Lunch	Snack	Dinner	Snack	Bedtime	Night	Notes
Blood Sugar									
Insulin Dose									
Grams Carb									
Activity									

Date:	Breakfast	Snack	Lunch	Snack	Dinner	Snack	Bedtime	Night	Notes
Blood Sugar									
Insulin Dose									
Grams Carb									
Activity									

Date:	Breakfast	Snack	Lunch	Snack	Dinner	Snack	Bedtime	Night	Notes
Blood Sugar									
Insulin Dose									
Grams Carb									
Activity									

Weekly Diabetes Record

Name: _____

Date:	Breakfast	Snack	Lunch	Snack	Dinner	Snack	Bedtime	Night	Notes
Blood Sugar									
Insulin Dose									
Grams Carb									
Activity									

Date:	Breakfast	Snack	Lunch	Snack	Dinner	Snack	Bedtime	Night	Notes
Blood Sugar									
Insulin Dose									
Grams Carb									
Activity									

Date:	Breakfast	Snack	Lunch	Snack	Dinner	Snack	Bedtime	Night	Notes
Blood Sugar									
Insulin Dose									
Grams Carb									
Activity									

Date:	Breakfast	Snack	Lunch	Snack	Dinner	Snack	Bedtime	Night	Notes
Blood Sugar									
Insulin Dose									
Grams Carb									
Activity									

Date:	Breakfast	Snack	Lunch	Snack	Dinner	Snack	Bedtime	Night	Notes
Blood Sugar									
Insulin Dose									
Grams Carb									
Activity									

Date:	Breakfast	Snack	Lunch	Snack	Dinner	Snack	Bedtime	Night	Notes
Blood Sugar									
Insulin Dose									
Grams Carb									
Activity									

Date:	Breakfast	Snack	Lunch	Snack	Dinner	Snack	Bedtime	Night	Notes
Blood Sugar									
Insulin Dose									
Grams Carb									
Activity									

Weekly Diabetes Record

Name:

Date:	Breakfast	Snack	Lunch	Snack	Dinner	Snack	Bedtime	Night	Notes
Blood Sugar									
Insulin Dose									
Grams Carb									
Activity									

Date:	Breakfast	Snack	Lunch	Snack	Dinner	Snack	Bedtime	Night	Notes
Blood Sugar									
Insulin Dose									
Grams Carb									
Activity									

Date:	Breakfast	Snack	Lunch	Snack	Dinner	Snack	Bedtime	Night	Notes
Blood Sugar									
Insulin Dose									
Grams Carb									
Activity									

Date:	Breakfast	Snack	Lunch	Snack	Dinner	Snack	Bedtime	Night	Notes
Blood Sugar									
Insulin Dose									
Grams Carb									
Activity									

Date:	Breakfast	Snack	Lunch	Snack	Dinner	Snack	Bedtime	Night	Notes
Blood Sugar									
Insulin Dose									
Grams Carb									
Activity									

Date:	Breakfast	Snack	Lunch	Snack	Dinner	Snack	Bedtime	Night	Notes
Blood Sugar									
Insulin Dose									
Grams Carb									
Activity									

Date:	Breakfast	Snack	Lunch	Snack	Dinner	Snack	Bedtime	Night	Notes
Blood Sugar									
Insulin Dose									
Grams Carb									
Activity									

Weekly Diabetes Record

Name:

Date:	Breakfast	Snack	Lunch	Snack	Dinner	Snack	Bedtime	Night	Notes
Blood Sugar									
Insulin Dose									
Grams Carb									
Activity									

Date:	Breakfast	Snack	Lunch	Snack	Dinner	Snack	Bedtime	Night	Notes
Blood Sugar									
Insulin Dose									
Grams Carb									
Activity									

Date:	Breakfast	Snack	Lunch	Snack	Dinner	Snack	Bedtime	Night	Notes
Blood Sugar									
Insulin Dose									
Grams Carb									
Activity									

Date:	Breakfast	Snack	Lunch	Snack	Dinner	Snack	Bedtime	Night	Notes
Blood Sugar									
Insulin Dose									
Grams Carb									
Activity									

Date:	Breakfast	Snack	Lunch	Snack	Dinner	Snack	Bedtime	Night	Notes
Blood Sugar									
Insulin Dose									
Grams Carb									
Activity									

Date:	Breakfast	Snack	Lunch	Snack	Dinner	Snack	Bedtime	Night	Notes
Blood Sugar									
Insulin Dose									
Grams Carb									
Activity									

Date:	Breakfast	Snack	Lunch	Snack	Dinner	Snack	Bedtime	Night	Notes
Blood Sugar									
Insulin Dose									
Grams Carb									
Activity									

Weekly Diabetes Record

Name: _____

Date:	Breakfast	Snack	Lunch	Snack	Dinner	Snack	Bedtime	Night	Notes
Blood Sugar									
Insulin Dose									
Grams Carb									
Activity									

Date:	Breakfast	Snack	Lunch	Snack	Dinner	Snack	Bedtime	Night	Notes
Blood Sugar									
Insulin Dose									
Grams Carb									
Activity									

Date:	Breakfast	Snack	Lunch	Snack	Dinner	Snack	Bedtime	Night	Notes
Blood Sugar									
Insulin Dose									
Grams Carb									
Activity									

Date:	Breakfast	Snack	Lunch	Snack	Dinner	Snack	Bedtime	Night	Notes
Blood Sugar									
Insulin Dose									
Grams Carb									
Activity									

Date:	Breakfast	Snack	Lunch	Snack	Dinner	Snack	Bedtime	Night	Notes
Blood Sugar									
Insulin Dose									
Grams Carb									
Activity									

Date:	Breakfast	Snack	Lunch	Snack	Dinner	Snack	Bedtime	Night	Notes
Blood Sugar									
Insulin Dose									
Grams Carb									
Activity									

Date:	Breakfast	Snack	Lunch	Snack	Dinner	Snack	Bedtime	Night	Notes
Blood Sugar									
Insulin Dose									
Grams Carb									
Activity									

Weekly Diabetes Record

Name:

Date:	Breakfast	Snack	Lunch	Snack	Dinner	Snack	Bedtime	Night	Notes
Blood Sugar									
Insulin Dose									
Grams Carb									
Activity									

Date:	Breakfast	Snack	Lunch	Snack	Dinner	Snack	Bedtime	Night	Notes
Blood Sugar									
Insulin Dose									
Grams Carb									
Activity									

Date:	Breakfast	Snack	Lunch	Snack	Dinner	Snack	Bedtime	Night	Notes
Blood Sugar									
Insulin Dose									
Grams Carb									
Activity									

Date:	Breakfast	Snack	Lunch	Snack	Dinner	Snack	Bedtime	Night	Notes
Blood Sugar									
Insulin Dose									
Grams Carb									
Activity									

Date:	Breakfast	Snack	Lunch	Snack	Dinner	Snack	Bedtime	Night	Notes
Blood Sugar									
Insulin Dose									
Grams Carb									
Activity									

Date:	Breakfast	Snack	Lunch	Snack	Dinner	Snack	Bedtime	Night	Notes
Blood Sugar									
Insulin Dose									
Grams Carb									
Activity									

Date:	Breakfast	Snack	Lunch	Snack	Dinner	Snack	Bedtime	Night	Notes
Blood Sugar									
Insulin Dose									
Grams Carb									
Activity									

Weekly Diabetes Record

Name:

Date:	Breakfast	Snack	Lunch	Snack	Dinner	Snack	Bedtime	Night	Notes
Blood Sugar									
Insulin Dose									
Grams Carb									
Activity									

Date:	Breakfast	Snack	Lunch	Snack	Dinner	Snack	Bedtime	Night	Notes
Blood Sugar									
Insulin Dose									
Grams Carb									
Activity									

Date:	Breakfast	Snack	Lunch	Snack	Dinner	Snack	Bedtime	Night	Notes
Blood Sugar									
Insulin Dose									
Grams Carb									
Activity									

Date:	Breakfast	Snack	Lunch	Snack	Dinner	Snack	Bedtime	Night	Notes
Blood Sugar									
Insulin Dose									
Grams Carb									
Activity									

Date:	Breakfast	Snack	Lunch	Snack	Dinner	Snack	Bedtime	Night	Notes
Blood Sugar									
Insulin Dose									
Grams Carb									
Activity									

Date:	Breakfast	Snack	Lunch	Snack	Dinner	Snack	Bedtime	Night	Notes
Blood Sugar									
Insulin Dose									
Grams Carb									
Activity									

Date:	Breakfast	Snack	Lunch	Snack	Dinner	Snack	Bedtime	Night	Notes
Blood Sugar									
Insulin Dose									
Grams Carb									
Activity									

Weekly Diabetes Record

Name: _____

Date:	Breakfast	Snack	Lunch	Snack	Dinner	Snack	Bedtime	Night	Notes
Blood Sugar									
Insulin Dose									
Grams Carb									
Activity									

Date:	Breakfast	Snack	Lunch	Snack	Dinner	Snack	Bedtime	Night	Notes
Blood Sugar									
Insulin Dose									
Grams Carb									
Activity									

Date:	Breakfast	Snack	Lunch	Snack	Dinner	Snack	Bedtime	Night	Notes
Blood Sugar									
Insulin Dose									
Grams Carb									
Activity									

Date:	Breakfast	Snack	Lunch	Snack	Dinner	Snack	Bedtime	Night	Notes
Blood Sugar									
Insulin Dose									
Grams Carb									
Activity									

Date:	Breakfast	Snack	Lunch	Snack	Dinner	Snack	Bedtime	Night	Notes
Blood Sugar									
Insulin Dose									
Grams Carb									
Activity									

Date:	Breakfast	Snack	Lunch	Snack	Dinner	Snack	Bedtime	Night	Notes
Blood Sugar									
Insulin Dose									
Grams Carb									
Activity									

Date:	Breakfast	Snack	Lunch	Snack	Dinner	Snack	Bedtime	Night	Notes
Blood Sugar									
Insulin Dose									
Grams Carb									
Activity									

Weekly Diabetes Record

Name:

Date:	Breakfast	Snack	Lunch	Snack	Dinner	Snack	Bedtime	Night	Notes
Blood Sugar									
Insulin Dose									
Grams Carb									
Activity									

Date:	Breakfast	Snack	Lunch	Snack	Dinner	Snack	Bedtime	Night	Notes
Blood Sugar									
Insulin Dose									
Grams Carb									
Activity									

Date:	Breakfast	Snack	Lunch	Snack	Dinner	Snack	Bedtime	Night	Notes
Blood Sugar									
Insulin Dose									
Grams Carb									
Activity									

Date:	Breakfast	Snack	Lunch	Snack	Dinner	Snack	Bedtime	Night	Notes
Blood Sugar									
Insulin Dose									
Grams Carb									
Activity									

Date:	Breakfast	Snack	Lunch	Snack	Dinner	Snack	Bedtime	Night	Notes
Blood Sugar									
Insulin Dose									
Grams Carb									
Activity									

Date:	Breakfast	Snack	Lunch	Snack	Dinner	Snack	Bedtime	Night	Notes
Blood Sugar									
Insulin Dose									
Grams Carb									
Activity									

Date:	Breakfast	Snack	Lunch	Snack	Dinner	Snack	Bedtime	Night	Notes
Blood Sugar									
Insulin Dose									
Grams Carb									
Activity									

Weekly Diabetes Record

Name: _____

Date:	Breakfast	Snack	Lunch	Snack	Dinner	Snack	Bedtime	Night	Notes
Blood Sugar									
Insulin Dose									
Grams Carb									
Activity									

Date:	Breakfast	Snack	Lunch	Snack	Dinner	Snack	Bedtime	Night	Notes
Blood Sugar									
Insulin Dose									
Grams Carb									
Activity									

Date:	Breakfast	Snack	Lunch	Snack	Dinner	Snack	Bedtime	Night	Notes
Blood Sugar									
Insulin Dose									
Grams Carb									
Activity									

Date:	Breakfast	Snack	Lunch	Snack	Dinner	Snack	Bedtime	Night	Notes
Blood Sugar									
Insulin Dose									
Grams Carb									
Activity									

Date:	Breakfast	Snack	Lunch	Snack	Dinner	Snack	Bedtime	Night	Notes
Blood Sugar									
Insulin Dose									
Grams Carb									
Activity									

Date:	Breakfast	Snack	Lunch	Snack	Dinner	Snack	Bedtime	Night	Notes
Blood Sugar									
Insulin Dose									
Grams Carb									
Activity									

Date:	Breakfast	Snack	Lunch	Snack	Dinner	Snack	Bedtime	Night	Notes
Blood Sugar									
Insulin Dose									
Grams Carb									
Activity									

Weekly Diabetes Record

Name: _____

Date:	Breakfast	Snack	Lunch	Snack	Dinner	Snack	Bedtime	Night	Notes
Blood Sugar									
Insulin Dose									
Grams Carb									
Activity									

Date:	Breakfast	Snack	Lunch	Snack	Dinner	Snack	Bedtime	Night	Notes
Blood Sugar									
Insulin Dose									
Grams Carb									
Activity									

Date:	Breakfast	Snack	Lunch	Snack	Dinner	Snack	Bedtime	Night	Notes
Blood Sugar									
Insulin Dose									
Grams Carb									
Activity									

Date:	Breakfast	Snack	Lunch	Snack	Dinner	Snack	Bedtime	Night	Notes
Blood Sugar									
Insulin Dose									
Grams Carb									
Activity									

Date:	Breakfast	Snack	Lunch	Snack	Dinner	Snack	Bedtime	Night	Notes
Blood Sugar									
Insulin Dose									
Grams Carb									
Activity									

Date:	Breakfast	Snack	Lunch	Snack	Dinner	Snack	Bedtime	Night	Notes
Blood Sugar									
Insulin Dose									
Grams Carb									
Activity									

Date:	Breakfast	Snack	Lunch	Snack	Dinner	Snack	Bedtime	Night	Notes
Blood Sugar									
Insulin Dose									
Grams Carb									
Activity									

Weekly Diabetes Record

Name: _____

Date:	Breakfast	Snack	Lunch	Snack	Dinner	Snack	Bedtime	Night	Notes
Blood Sugar									
Insulin Dose									
Grams Carb									
Activity									

Date:	Breakfast	Snack	Lunch	Snack	Dinner	Snack	Bedtime	Night	Notes
Blood Sugar									
Insulin Dose									
Grams Carb									
Activity									

Date:	Breakfast	Snack	Lunch	Snack	Dinner	Snack	Bedtime	Night	Notes
Blood Sugar									
Insulin Dose									
Grams Carb									
Activity									

Date:	Breakfast	Snack	Lunch	Snack	Dinner	Snack	Bedtime	Night	Notes
Blood Sugar									
Insulin Dose									
Grams Carb									
Activity									

Date:	Breakfast	Snack	Lunch	Snack	Dinner	Snack	Bedtime	Night	Notes
Blood Sugar									
Insulin Dose									
Grams Carb									
Activity									

Date:	Breakfast	Snack	Lunch	Snack	Dinner	Snack	Bedtime	Night	Notes
Blood Sugar									
Insulin Dose									
Grams Carb									
Activity									

Date:	Breakfast	Snack	Lunch	Snack	Dinner	Snack	Bedtime	Night	Notes
Blood Sugar									
Insulin Dose									
Grams Carb									
Activity									

Weekly Diabetes Record

Name:

Date:	Breakfast	Snack	Lunch	Snack	Dinner	Snack	Bedtime	Night	Notes
Blood Sugar									
Insulin Dose									
Grams Carb									
Activity									

Date:	Breakfast	Snack	Lunch	Snack	Dinner	Snack	Bedtime	Night	Notes
Blood Sugar									
Insulin Dose									
Grams Carb									
Activity									

Date:	Breakfast	Snack	Lunch	Snack	Dinner	Snack	Bedtime	Night	Notes
Blood Sugar									
Insulin Dose									
Grams Carb									
Activity									

Date:	Breakfast	Snack	Lunch	Snack	Dinner	Snack	Bedtime	Night	Notes
Blood Sugar									
Insulin Dose									
Grams Carb									
Activity									

Date:	Breakfast	Snack	Lunch	Snack	Dinner	Snack	Bedtime	Night	Notes
Blood Sugar									
Insulin Dose									
Grams Carb									
Activity									

Date:	Breakfast	Snack	Lunch	Snack	Dinner	Snack	Bedtime	Night	Notes
Blood Sugar									
Insulin Dose									
Grams Carb									
Activity									

Date:	Breakfast	Snack	Lunch	Snack	Dinner	Snack	Bedtime	Night	Notes
Blood Sugar									
Insulin Dose									
Grams Carb									
Activity									

Weekly Diabetes Record

Name: _____

Date:	Breakfast	Snack	Lunch	Snack	Dinner	Snack	Bedtime	Night	Notes
Blood Sugar									
Insulin Dose									
Grams Carb									
Activity									

Date:	Breakfast	Snack	Lunch	Snack	Dinner	Snack	Bedtime	Night	Notes
Blood Sugar									
Insulin Dose									
Grams Carb									
Activity									

Date:	Breakfast	Snack	Lunch	Snack	Dinner	Snack	Bedtime	Night	Notes
Blood Sugar									
Insulin Dose									
Grams Carb									
Activity									

Date:	Breakfast	Snack	Lunch	Snack	Dinner	Snack	Bedtime	Night	Notes
Blood Sugar									
Insulin Dose									
Grams Carb									
Activity									

Date:	Breakfast	Snack	Lunch	Snack	Dinner	Snack	Bedtime	Night	Notes
Blood Sugar									
Insulin Dose									
Grams Carb									
Activity									

Date:	Breakfast	Snack	Lunch	Snack	Dinner	Snack	Bedtime	Night	Notes
Blood Sugar									
Insulin Dose									
Grams Carb									
Activity									

Date:	Breakfast	Snack	Lunch	Snack	Dinner	Snack	Bedtime	Night	Notes
Blood Sugar									
Insulin Dose									
Grams Carb									
Activity									

Weekly Diabetes Record

Name: _____

Date:	Breakfast	Snack	Lunch	Snack	Dinner	Snack	Bedtime	Night	Notes
Blood Sugar									
Insulin Dose									
Grams Carb									
Activity									

Date:	Breakfast	Snack	Lunch	Snack	Dinner	Snack	Bedtime	Night	Notes
Blood Sugar									
Insulin Dose									
Grams Carb									
Activity									

Date:	Breakfast	Snack	Lunch	Snack	Dinner	Snack	Bedtime	Night	Notes
Blood Sugar									
Insulin Dose									
Grams Carb									
Activity									

Date:	Breakfast	Snack	Lunch	Snack	Dinner	Snack	Bedtime	Night	Notes
Blood Sugar									
Insulin Dose									
Grams Carb									
Activity									

Date:	Breakfast	Snack	Lunch	Snack	Dinner	Snack	Bedtime	Night	Notes
Blood Sugar									
Insulin Dose									
Grams Carb									
Activity									

Date:	Breakfast	Snack	Lunch	Snack	Dinner	Snack	Bedtime	Night	Notes
Blood Sugar									
Insulin Dose									
Grams Carb									
Activity									

Date:	Breakfast	Snack	Lunch	Snack	Dinner	Snack	Bedtime	Night	Notes
Blood Sugar									
Insulin Dose									
Grams Carb									
Activity									

Weekly Diabetes Record

Name: _____

Date:	Breakfast	Snack	Lunch	Snack	Dinner	Snack	Bedtime	Night	Notes
Blood Sugar									
Insulin Dose									
Grams Carb									
Activity									

Date:	Breakfast	Snack	Lunch	Snack	Dinner	Snack	Bedtime	Night	Notes
Blood Sugar									
Insulin Dose									
Grams Carb									
Activity									

Date:	Breakfast	Snack	Lunch	Snack	Dinner	Snack	Bedtime	Night	Notes
Blood Sugar									
Insulin Dose									
Grams Carb									
Activity									

Date:	Breakfast	Snack	Lunch	Snack	Dinner	Snack	Bedtime	Night	Notes
Blood Sugar									
Insulin Dose									
Grams Carb									
Activity									

Date:	Breakfast	Snack	Lunch	Snack	Dinner	Snack	Bedtime	Night	Notes
Blood Sugar									
Insulin Dose									
Grams Carb									
Activity									

Date:	Breakfast	Snack	Lunch	Snack	Dinner	Snack	Bedtime	Night	Notes
Blood Sugar									
Insulin Dose									
Grams Carb									
Activity									

Date:	Breakfast	Snack	Lunch	Snack	Dinner	Snack	Bedtime	Night	Notes
Blood Sugar									
Insulin Dose									
Grams Carb									
Activity									

Weekly Diabetes Record

Name:

Date:	Breakfast	Snack	Lunch	Snack	Dinner	Snack	Bedtime	Night	Notes
Blood Sugar									
Insulin Dose									
Grams Carb									
Activity									

Date:	Breakfast	Snack	Lunch	Snack	Dinner	Snack	Bedtime	Night	Notes
Blood Sugar									
Insulin Dose									
Grams Carb									
Activity									

Date:	Breakfast	Snack	Lunch	Snack	Dinner	Snack	Bedtime	Night	Notes
Blood Sugar									
Insulin Dose									
Grams Carb									
Activity									

Date:	Breakfast	Snack	Lunch	Snack	Dinner	Snack	Bedtime	Night	Notes
Blood Sugar									
Insulin Dose									
Grams Carb									
Activity									

Date:	Breakfast	Snack	Lunch	Snack	Dinner	Snack	Bedtime	Night	Notes
Blood Sugar									
Insulin Dose									
Grams Carb									
Activity									

Date:	Breakfast	Snack	Lunch	Snack	Dinner	Snack	Bedtime	Night	Notes
Blood Sugar									
Insulin Dose									
Grams Carb									
Activity									

Date:	Breakfast	Snack	Lunch	Snack	Dinner	Snack	Bedtime	Night	Notes
Blood Sugar									
Insulin Dose									
Grams Carb									
Activity									

Weekly Diabetes Record

Name: _____

Date:	Breakfast	Snack	Lunch	Snack	Dinner	Snack	Bedtime	Night	Notes
Blood Sugar									
Insulin Dose									
Grams Carb									
Activity									

Date:	Breakfast	Snack	Lunch	Snack	Dinner	Snack	Bedtime	Night	Notes
Blood Sugar									
Insulin Dose									
Grams Carb									
Activity									

Date:	Breakfast	Snack	Lunch	Snack	Dinner	Snack	Bedtime	Night	Notes
Blood Sugar									
Insulin Dose									
Grams Carb									
Activity									

Date:	Breakfast	Snack	Lunch	Snack	Dinner	Snack	Bedtime	Night	Notes
Blood Sugar									
Insulin Dose									
Grams Carb									
Activity									

Date:	Breakfast	Snack	Lunch	Snack	Dinner	Snack	Bedtime	Night	Notes
Blood Sugar									
Insulin Dose									
Grams Carb									
Activity									

Date:	Breakfast	Snack	Lunch	Snack	Dinner	Snack	Bedtime	Night	Notes
Blood Sugar									
Insulin Dose									
Grams Carb									
Activity									

Date:	Breakfast	Snack	Lunch	Snack	Dinner	Snack	Bedtime	Night	Notes
Blood Sugar									
Insulin Dose									
Grams Carb									
Activity									

Weekly Diabetes Record

Name:

Date:	Breakfast	Snack	Lunch	Snack	Dinner	Snack	Bedtime	Night	Notes
Blood Sugar									
Insulin Dose									
Grams Carb									
Activity									

Date:	Breakfast	Snack	Lunch	Snack	Dinner	Snack	Bedtime	Night	Notes
Blood Sugar									
Insulin Dose									
Grams Carb									
Activity									

Date:	Breakfast	Snack	Lunch	Snack	Dinner	Snack	Bedtime	Night	Notes
Blood Sugar									
Insulin Dose									
Grams Carb									
Activity									

Date:	Breakfast	Snack	Lunch	Snack	Dinner	Snack	Bedtime	Night	Notes
Blood Sugar									
Insulin Dose									
Grams Carb									
Activity									

Date:	Breakfast	Snack	Lunch	Snack	Dinner	Snack	Bedtime	Night	Notes
Blood Sugar									
Insulin Dose									
Grams Carb									
Activity									

Date:	Breakfast	Snack	Lunch	Snack	Dinner	Snack	Bedtime	Night	Notes
Blood Sugar									
Insulin Dose									
Grams Carb									
Activity									

Date:	Breakfast	Snack	Lunch	Snack	Dinner	Snack	Bedtime	Night	Notes
Blood Sugar									
Insulin Dose									
Grams Carb									
Activity									

Weekly Diabetes Record

Name: _____

Date:	Breakfast	Snack	Lunch	Snack	Dinner	Snack	Bedtime	Night	Notes
Blood Sugar									
Insulin Dose									
Grams Carb									
Activity									

Date:	Breakfast	Snack	Lunch	Snack	Dinner	Snack	Bedtime	Night	Notes
Blood Sugar									
Insulin Dose									
Grams Carb									
Activity									

Date:	Breakfast	Snack	Lunch	Snack	Dinner	Snack	Bedtime	Night	Notes
Blood Sugar									
Insulin Dose									
Grams Carb									
Activity									

Date:	Breakfast	Snack	Lunch	Snack	Dinner	Snack	Bedtime	Night	Notes
Blood Sugar									
Insulin Dose									
Grams Carb									
Activity									

Date:	Breakfast	Snack	Lunch	Snack	Dinner	Snack	Bedtime	Night	Notes
Blood Sugar									
Insulin Dose									
Grams Carb									
Activity									

Date:	Breakfast	Snack	Lunch	Snack	Dinner	Snack	Bedtime	Night	Notes
Blood Sugar									
Insulin Dose									
Grams Carb									
Activity									

Date:	Breakfast	Snack	Lunch	Snack	Dinner	Snack	Bedtime	Night	Notes
Blood Sugar									
Insulin Dose									
Grams Carb									
Activity									

Weekly Diabetes Record

Name:

Date:	Breakfast	Snack	Lunch	Snack	Dinner	Snack	Bedtime	Night	Notes
Blood Sugar									
Insulin Dose									
Grams Carb									
Activity									

Date:	Breakfast	Snack	Lunch	Snack	Dinner	Snack	Bedtime	Night	Notes
Blood Sugar									
Insulin Dose									
Grams Carb									
Activity									

Date:	Breakfast	Snack	Lunch	Snack	Dinner	Snack	Bedtime	Night	Notes
Blood Sugar									
Insulin Dose									
Grams Carb									
Activity									

Date:	Breakfast	Snack	Lunch	Snack	Dinner	Snack	Bedtime	Night	Notes
Blood Sugar									
Insulin Dose									
Grams Carb									
Activity									

Date:	Breakfast	Snack	Lunch	Snack	Dinner	Snack	Bedtime	Night	Notes
Blood Sugar									
Insulin Dose									
Grams Carb									
Activity									

Date:	Breakfast	Snack	Lunch	Snack	Dinner	Snack	Bedtime	Night	Notes
Blood Sugar									
Insulin Dose									
Grams Carb									
Activity									

Date:	Breakfast	Snack	Lunch	Snack	Dinner	Snack	Bedtime	Night	Notes
Blood Sugar									
Insulin Dose									
Grams Carb									
Activity									

Weekly Diabetes Record

Name: _____

Date:	Breakfast	Snack	Lunch	Snack	Dinner	Snack	Bedtime	Night	Notes
Blood Sugar									
Insulin Dose									
Grams Carb									
Activity									

Date:	Breakfast	Snack	Lunch	Snack	Dinner	Snack	Bedtime	Night	Notes
Blood Sugar									
Insulin Dose									
Grams Carb									
Activity									

Date:	Breakfast	Snack	Lunch	Snack	Dinner	Snack	Bedtime	Night	Notes
Blood Sugar									
Insulin Dose									
Grams Carb									
Activity									

Date:	Breakfast	Snack	Lunch	Snack	Dinner	Snack	Bedtime	Night	Notes
Blood Sugar									
Insulin Dose									
Grams Carb									
Activity									

Date:	Breakfast	Snack	Lunch	Snack	Dinner	Snack	Bedtime	Night	Notes
Blood Sugar									
Insulin Dose									
Grams Carb									
Activity									

Date:	Breakfast	Snack	Lunch	Snack	Dinner	Snack	Bedtime	Night	Notes
Blood Sugar									
Insulin Dose									
Grams Carb									
Activity									

Date:	Breakfast	Snack	Lunch	Snack	Dinner	Snack	Bedtime	Night	Notes
Blood Sugar									
Insulin Dose									
Grams Carb									
Activity									

Weekly Diabetes Record

Name: _____

Date:	Breakfast	Snack	Lunch	Snack	Dinner	Snack	Bedtime	Night	Notes
Blood Sugar									
Insulin Dose									
Grams Carb									
Activity									

Date:	Breakfast	Snack	Lunch	Snack	Dinner	Snack	Bedtime	Night	Notes
Blood Sugar									
Insulin Dose									
Grams Carb									
Activity									

Date:	Breakfast	Snack	Lunch	Snack	Dinner	Snack	Bedtime	Night	Notes
Blood Sugar									
Insulin Dose									
Grams Carb									
Activity									

Date:	Breakfast	Snack	Lunch	Snack	Dinner	Snack	Bedtime	Night	Notes
Blood Sugar									
Insulin Dose									
Grams Carb									
Activity									

Date:	Breakfast	Snack	Lunch	Snack	Dinner	Snack	Bedtime	Night	Notes
Blood Sugar									
Insulin Dose									
Grams Carb									
Activity									

Date:	Breakfast	Snack	Lunch	Snack	Dinner	Snack	Bedtime	Night	Notes
Blood Sugar									
Insulin Dose									
Grams Carb									
Activity									

Date:	Breakfast	Snack	Lunch	Snack	Dinner	Snack	Bedtime	Night	Notes
Blood Sugar									
Insulin Dose									
Grams Carb									
Activity									

Weekly Diabetes Record

Name: _____

Date:	Breakfast	Snack	Lunch	Snack	Dinner	Snack	Bedtime	Night	Notes
Blood Sugar									
Insulin Dose									
Grams Carb									
Activity									

Date:	Breakfast	Snack	Lunch	Snack	Dinner	Snack	Bedtime	Night	Notes
Blood Sugar									
Insulin Dose									
Grams Carb									
Activity									

Date:	Breakfast	Snack	Lunch	Snack	Dinner	Snack	Bedtime	Night	Notes
Blood Sugar									
Insulin Dose									
Grams Carb									
Activity									

Date:	Breakfast	Snack	Lunch	Snack	Dinner	Snack	Bedtime	Night	Notes
Blood Sugar									
Insulin Dose									
Grams Carb									
Activity									

Date:	Breakfast	Snack	Lunch	Snack	Dinner	Snack	Bedtime	Night	Notes
Blood Sugar									
Insulin Dose									
Grams Carb									
Activity									

Date:	Breakfast	Snack	Lunch	Snack	Dinner	Snack	Bedtime	Night	Notes
Blood Sugar									
Insulin Dose									
Grams Carb									
Activity									

Date:	Breakfast	Snack	Lunch	Snack	Dinner	Snack	Bedtime	Night	Notes
Blood Sugar									
Insulin Dose									
Grams Carb									
Activity									

Weekly Diabetes Record

Name: _____

Date:	Breakfast	Snack	Lunch	Snack	Dinner	Snack	Bedtime	Night	Notes
Blood Sugar									
Insulin Dose									
Grams Carb									
Activity									

Date:	Breakfast	Snack	Lunch	Snack	Dinner	Snack	Bedtime	Night	Notes
Blood Sugar									
Insulin Dose									
Grams Carb									
Activity									

Date:	Breakfast	Snack	Lunch	Snack	Dinner	Snack	Bedtime	Night	Notes
Blood Sugar									
Insulin Dose									
Grams Carb									
Activity									

Date:	Breakfast	Snack	Lunch	Snack	Dinner	Snack	Bedtime	Night	Notes
Blood Sugar									
Insulin Dose									
Grams Carb									
Activity									

Date:	Breakfast	Snack	Lunch	Snack	Dinner	Snack	Bedtime	Night	Notes
Blood Sugar									
Insulin Dose									
Grams Carb									
Activity									

Date:	Breakfast	Snack	Lunch	Snack	Dinner	Snack	Bedtime	Night	Notes
Blood Sugar									
Insulin Dose									
Grams Carb									
Activity									

Date:	Breakfast	Snack	Lunch	Snack	Dinner	Snack	Bedtime	Night	Notes
Blood Sugar									
Insulin Dose									
Grams Carb									
Activity									

Weekly Diabetes Record

Name: _____

Date:	Breakfast	Snack	Lunch	Snack	Dinner	Snack	Bedtime	Night	Notes
Blood Sugar									
Insulin Dose									
Grams Carb									
Activity									

Date:	Breakfast	Snack	Lunch	Snack	Dinner	Snack	Bedtime	Night	Notes
Blood Sugar									
Insulin Dose									
Grams Carb									
Activity									

Date:	Breakfast	Snack	Lunch	Snack	Dinner	Snack	Bedtime	Night	Notes
Blood Sugar									
Insulin Dose									
Grams Carb									
Activity									

Date:	Breakfast	Snack	Lunch	Snack	Dinner	Snack	Bedtime	Night	Notes
Blood Sugar									
Insulin Dose									
Grams Carb									
Activity									

Date:	Breakfast	Snack	Lunch	Snack	Dinner	Snack	Bedtime	Night	Notes
Blood Sugar									
Insulin Dose									
Grams Carb									
Activity									

Date:	Breakfast	Snack	Lunch	Snack	Dinner	Snack	Bedtime	Night	Notes
Blood Sugar									
Insulin Dose									
Grams Carb									
Activity									

Date:	Breakfast	Snack	Lunch	Snack	Dinner	Snack	Bedtime	Night	Notes
Blood Sugar									
Insulin Dose									
Grams Carb									
Activity									

Weekly Diabetes Record

Name:

Date:	Breakfast	Snack	Lunch	Snack	Dinner	Snack	Bedtime	Night	Notes
Blood Sugar									
Insulin Dose									
Grams Carb									
Activity									

Date:	Breakfast	Snack	Lunch	Snack	Dinner	Snack	Bedtime	Night	Notes
Blood Sugar									
Insulin Dose									
Grams Carb									
Activity									

Date:	Breakfast	Snack	Lunch	Snack	Dinner	Snack	Bedtime	Night	Notes
Blood Sugar									
Insulin Dose									
Grams Carb									
Activity									

Date:	Breakfast	Snack	Lunch	Snack	Dinner	Snack	Bedtime	Night	Notes
Blood Sugar									
Insulin Dose									
Grams Carb									
Activity									

Date:	Breakfast	Snack	Lunch	Snack	Dinner	Snack	Bedtime	Night	Notes
Blood Sugar									
Insulin Dose									
Grams Carb									
Activity									

Date:	Breakfast	Snack	Lunch	Snack	Dinner	Snack	Bedtime	Night	Notes
Blood Sugar									
Insulin Dose									
Grams Carb									
Activity									

Date:	Breakfast	Snack	Lunch	Snack	Dinner	Snack	Bedtime	Night	Notes
Blood Sugar									
Insulin Dose									
Grams Carb									
Activity									

Weekly Diabetes Record

Name: _____

Date:	Breakfast	Snack	Lunch	Snack	Dinner	Snack	Bedtime	Night	Notes
Blood Sugar									
Insulin Dose									
Grams Carb									
Activity									

Date:	Breakfast	Snack	Lunch	Snack	Dinner	Snack	Bedtime	Night	Notes
Blood Sugar									
Insulin Dose									
Grams Carb									
Activity									

Date:	Breakfast	Snack	Lunch	Snack	Dinner	Snack	Bedtime	Night	Notes
Blood Sugar									
Insulin Dose									
Grams Carb									
Activity									

Date:	Breakfast	Snack	Lunch	Snack	Dinner	Snack	Bedtime	Night	Notes
Blood Sugar									
Insulin Dose									
Grams Carb									
Activity									

Date:	Breakfast	Snack	Lunch	Snack	Dinner	Snack	Bedtime	Night	Notes
Blood Sugar									
Insulin Dose									
Grams Carb									
Activity									

Date:	Breakfast	Snack	Lunch	Snack	Dinner	Snack	Bedtime	Night	Notes
Blood Sugar									
Insulin Dose									
Grams Carb									
Activity									

Date:	Breakfast	Snack	Lunch	Snack	Dinner	Snack	Bedtime	Night	Notes
Blood Sugar									
Insulin Dose									
Grams Carb									
Activity									

Weekly Diabetes Record

Name:

Date:	Breakfast	Snack	Lunch	Snack	Dinner	Snack	Bedtime	Night	Notes
Blood Sugar									
Insulin Dose									
Grams Carb									
Activity									

Date:	Breakfast	Snack	Lunch	Snack	Dinner	Snack	Bedtime	Night	Notes
Blood Sugar									
Insulin Dose									
Grams Carb									
Activity									

Date:	Breakfast	Snack	Lunch	Snack	Dinner	Snack	Bedtime	Night	Notes
Blood Sugar									
Insulin Dose									
Grams Carb									
Activity									

Date:	Breakfast	Snack	Lunch	Snack	Dinner	Snack	Bedtime	Night	Notes
Blood Sugar									
Insulin Dose									
Grams Carb									
Activity									

Date:	Breakfast	Snack	Lunch	Snack	Dinner	Snack	Bedtime	Night	Notes
Blood Sugar									
Insulin Dose									
Grams Carb									
Activity									

Date:	Breakfast	Snack	Lunch	Snack	Dinner	Snack	Bedtime	Night	Notes
Blood Sugar									
Insulin Dose									
Grams Carb									
Activity									

Date:	Breakfast	Snack	Lunch	Snack	Dinner	Snack	Bedtime	Night	Notes
Blood Sugar									
Insulin Dose									
Grams Carb									
Activity									

Weekly Diabetes Record

Name:

Date:	Breakfast	Snack	Lunch	Snack	Dinner	Snack	Bedtime	Night	Notes
Blood Sugar									
Insulin Dose									
Grams Carb									
Activity									

Date:	Breakfast	Snack	Lunch	Snack	Dinner	Snack	Bedtime	Night	Notes
Blood Sugar									
Insulin Dose									
Grams Carb									
Activity									

Date:	Breakfast	Snack	Lunch	Snack	Dinner	Snack	Bedtime	Night	Notes
Blood Sugar									
Insulin Dose									
Grams Carb									
Activity									

Date:	Breakfast	Snack	Lunch	Snack	Dinner	Snack	Bedtime	Night	Notes
Blood Sugar									
Insulin Dose									
Grams Carb									
Activity									

Date:	Breakfast	Snack	Lunch	Snack	Dinner	Snack	Bedtime	Night	Notes
Blood Sugar									
Insulin Dose									
Grams Carb									
Activity									

Date:	Breakfast	Snack	Lunch	Snack	Dinner	Snack	Bedtime	Night	Notes
Blood Sugar									
Insulin Dose									
Grams Carb									
Activity									

Date:	Breakfast	Snack	Lunch	Snack	Dinner	Snack	Bedtime	Night	Notes
Blood Sugar									
Insulin Dose									
Grams Carb									
Activity									

Weekly Diabetes Record

Name:

Date:	Breakfast	Snack	Lunch	Snack	Dinner	Snack	Bedtime	Night	Notes
Blood Sugar									
Insulin Dose									
Grams Carb									
Activity									

Date:	Breakfast	Snack	Lunch	Snack	Dinner	Snack	Bedtime	Night	Notes
Blood Sugar									
Insulin Dose									
Grams Carb									
Activity									

Date:	Breakfast	Snack	Lunch	Snack	Dinner	Snack	Bedtime	Night	Notes
Blood Sugar									
Insulin Dose									
Grams Carb									
Activity									

Date:	Breakfast	Snack	Lunch	Snack	Dinner	Snack	Bedtime	Night	Notes
Blood Sugar									
Insulin Dose									
Grams Carb									
Activity									

Date:	Breakfast	Snack	Lunch	Snack	Dinner	Snack	Bedtime	Night	Notes
Blood Sugar									
Insulin Dose									
Grams Carb									
Activity									

Date:	Breakfast	Snack	Lunch	Snack	Dinner	Snack	Bedtime	Night	Notes
Blood Sugar									
Insulin Dose									
Grams Carb									
Activity									

Date:	Breakfast	Snack	Lunch	Snack	Dinner	Snack	Bedtime	Night	Notes
Blood Sugar									
Insulin Dose									
Grams Carb									
Activity									

Weekly Diabetes Record

Name: _____

Date:	Breakfast	Snack	Lunch	Snack	Dinner	Snack	Bedtime	Night	Notes
Blood Sugar									
Insulin Dose									
Grams Carb									
Activity									

Date:	Breakfast	Snack	Lunch	Snack	Dinner	Snack	Bedtime	Night	Notes
Blood Sugar									
Insulin Dose									
Grams Carb									
Activity									

Date:	Breakfast	Snack	Lunch	Snack	Dinner	Snack	Bedtime	Night	Notes
Blood Sugar									
Insulin Dose									
Grams Carb									
Activity									

Date:	Breakfast	Snack	Lunch	Snack	Dinner	Snack	Bedtime	Night	Notes
Blood Sugar									
Insulin Dose									
Grams Carb									
Activity									

Date:	Breakfast	Snack	Lunch	Snack	Dinner	Snack	Bedtime	Night	Notes
Blood Sugar									
Insulin Dose									
Grams Carb									
Activity									

Date:	Breakfast	Snack	Lunch	Snack	Dinner	Snack	Bedtime	Night	Notes
Blood Sugar									
Insulin Dose									
Grams Carb									
Activity									

Date:	Breakfast	Snack	Lunch	Snack	Dinner	Snack	Bedtime	Night	Notes
Blood Sugar									
Insulin Dose									
Grams Carb									
Activity									

Weekly Diabetes Record

Name:

Date:	Breakfast	Snack	Lunch	Snack	Dinner	Snack	Bedtime	Night	Notes
Blood Sugar									
Insulin Dose									
Grams Carb									
Activity									

Date:	Breakfast	Snack	Lunch	Snack	Dinner	Snack	Bedtime	Night	Notes
Blood Sugar									
Insulin Dose									
Grams Carb									
Activity									

Date:	Breakfast	Snack	Lunch	Snack	Dinner	Snack	Bedtime	Night	Notes
Blood Sugar									
Insulin Dose									
Grams Carb									
Activity									

Date:	Breakfast	Snack	Lunch	Snack	Dinner	Snack	Bedtime	Night	Notes
Blood Sugar									
Insulin Dose									
Grams Carb									
Activity									

Date:	Breakfast	Snack	Lunch	Snack	Dinner	Snack	Bedtime	Night	Notes
Blood Sugar									
Insulin Dose									
Grams Carb									
Activity									

Date:	Breakfast	Snack	Lunch	Snack	Dinner	Snack	Bedtime	Night	Notes
Blood Sugar									
Insulin Dose									
Grams Carb									
Activity									

Date:	Breakfast	Snack	Lunch	Snack	Dinner	Snack	Bedtime	Night	Notes
Blood Sugar									
Insulin Dose									
Grams Carb									
Activity									

Weekly Diabetes Record

Name: _____

Date:	Breakfast	Snack	Lunch	Snack	Dinner	Snack	Bedtime	Night	Notes
Blood Sugar									
Insulin Dose									
Grams Carb									
Activity									

Date:	Breakfast	Snack	Lunch	Snack	Dinner	Snack	Bedtime	Night	Notes
Blood Sugar									
Insulin Dose									
Grams Carb									
Activity									

Date:	Breakfast	Snack	Lunch	Snack	Dinner	Snack	Bedtime	Night	Notes
Blood Sugar									
Insulin Dose									
Grams Carb									
Activity									

Date:	Breakfast	Snack	Lunch	Snack	Dinner	Snack	Bedtime	Night	Notes
Blood Sugar									
Insulin Dose									
Grams Carb									
Activity									

Date:	Breakfast	Snack	Lunch	Snack	Dinner	Snack	Bedtime	Night	Notes
Blood Sugar									
Insulin Dose									
Grams Carb									
Activity									

Date:	Breakfast	Snack	Lunch	Snack	Dinner	Snack	Bedtime	Night	Notes
Blood Sugar									
Insulin Dose									
Grams Carb									
Activity									

Date:	Breakfast	Snack	Lunch	Snack	Dinner	Snack	Bedtime	Night	Notes
Blood Sugar									
Insulin Dose									
Grams Carb									
Activity									

Weekly Diabetes Record

Name:

Date:	Breakfast	Snack	Lunch	Snack	Dinner	Snack	Bedtime	Night	Notes
Blood Sugar									
Insulin Dose									
Grams Carb									
Activity									

Date:	Breakfast	Snack	Lunch	Snack	Dinner	Snack	Bedtime	Night	Notes
Blood Sugar									
Insulin Dose									
Grams Carb									
Activity									

Date:	Breakfast	Snack	Lunch	Snack	Dinner	Snack	Bedtime	Night	Notes
Blood Sugar									
Insulin Dose									
Grams Carb									
Activity									

Date:	Breakfast	Snack	Lunch	Snack	Dinner	Snack	Bedtime	Night	Notes
Blood Sugar									
Insulin Dose									
Grams Carb									
Activity									

Date:	Breakfast	Snack	Lunch	Snack	Dinner	Snack	Bedtime	Night	Notes
Blood Sugar									
Insulin Dose									
Grams Carb									
Activity									

Date:	Breakfast	Snack	Lunch	Snack	Dinner	Snack	Bedtime	Night	Notes
Blood Sugar									
Insulin Dose									
Grams Carb									
Activity									

Date:	Breakfast	Snack	Lunch	Snack	Dinner	Snack	Bedtime	Night	Notes
Blood Sugar									
Insulin Dose									
Grams Carb									
Activity									

Weekly Diabetes Record

Name:

Date:	Breakfast	Snack	Lunch	Snack	Dinner	Snack	Bedtime	Night	Notes
Blood Sugar									
Insulin Dose									
Grams Carb									
Activity									

Date:	Breakfast	Snack	Lunch	Snack	Dinner	Snack	Bedtime	Night	Notes
Blood Sugar									
Insulin Dose									
Grams Carb									
Activity									

Date:	Breakfast	Snack	Lunch	Snack	Dinner	Snack	Bedtime	Night	Notes
Blood Sugar									
Insulin Dose									
Grams Carb									
Activity									

Date:	Breakfast	Snack	Lunch	Snack	Dinner	Snack	Bedtime	Night	Notes
Blood Sugar									
Insulin Dose									
Grams Carb									
Activity									

Date:	Breakfast	Snack	Lunch	Snack	Dinner	Snack	Bedtime	Night	Notes
Blood Sugar									
Insulin Dose									
Grams Carb									
Activity									

Date:	Breakfast	Snack	Lunch	Snack	Dinner	Snack	Bedtime	Night	Notes
Blood Sugar									
Insulin Dose									
Grams Carb									
Activity									

Date:	Breakfast	Snack	Lunch	Snack	Dinner	Snack	Bedtime	Night	Notes
Blood Sugar									
Insulin Dose									
Grams Carb									
Activity									

Weekly Diabetes Record

Name:

Date:	Breakfast	Snack	Lunch	Snack	Dinner	Snack	Bedtime	Night	Notes
Blood Sugar									
Insulin Dose									
Grams Carb									
Activity									

Date:	Breakfast	Snack	Lunch	Snack	Dinner	Snack	Bedtime	Night	Notes
Blood Sugar									
Insulin Dose									
Grams Carb									
Activity									

Date:	Breakfast	Snack	Lunch	Snack	Dinner	Snack	Bedtime	Night	Notes
Blood Sugar									
Insulin Dose									
Grams Carb									
Activity									

Date:	Breakfast	Snack	Lunch	Snack	Dinner	Snack	Bedtime	Night	Notes
Blood Sugar									
Insulin Dose									
Grams Carb									
Activity									

Date:	Breakfast	Snack	Lunch	Snack	Dinner	Snack	Bedtime	Night	Notes
Blood Sugar									
Insulin Dose									
Grams Carb									
Activity									

Date:	Breakfast	Snack	Lunch	Snack	Dinner	Snack	Bedtime	Night	Notes
Blood Sugar									
Insulin Dose									
Grams Carb									
Activity									

Date:	Breakfast	Snack	Lunch	Snack	Dinner	Snack	Bedtime	Night	Notes
Blood Sugar									
Insulin Dose									
Grams Carb									
Activity									

Weekly Diabetes Record

Name: _____

Date:	Breakfast	Snack	Lunch	Snack	Dinner	Snack	Bedtime	Night	Notes
Blood Sugar									
Insulin Dose									
Grams Carb									
Activity									

Date:	Breakfast	Snack	Lunch	Snack	Dinner	Snack	Bedtime	Night	Notes
Blood Sugar									
Insulin Dose									
Grams Carb									
Activity									

Date:	Breakfast	Snack	Lunch	Snack	Dinner	Snack	Bedtime	Night	Notes
Blood Sugar									
Insulin Dose									
Grams Carb									
Activity									

Date:	Breakfast	Snack	Lunch	Snack	Dinner	Snack	Bedtime	Night	Notes
Blood Sugar									
Insulin Dose									
Grams Carb									
Activity									

Date:	Breakfast	Snack	Lunch	Snack	Dinner	Snack	Bedtime	Night	Notes
Blood Sugar									
Insulin Dose									
Grams Carb									
Activity									

Date:	Breakfast	Snack	Lunch	Snack	Dinner	Snack	Bedtime	Night	Notes
Blood Sugar									
Insulin Dose									
Grams Carb									
Activity									

Date:	Breakfast	Snack	Lunch	Snack	Dinner	Snack	Bedtime	Night	Notes
Blood Sugar									
Insulin Dose									
Grams Carb									
Activity									

Weekly Diabetes Record

Name:

Date:	Breakfast	Snack	Lunch	Snack	Dinner	Snack	Bedtime	Night	Notes
Blood Sugar									
Insulin Dose									
Grams Carb									
Activity									

Date:	Breakfast	Snack	Lunch	Snack	Dinner	Snack	Bedtime	Night	Notes
Blood Sugar									
Insulin Dose									
Grams Carb									
Activity									

Date:	Breakfast	Snack	Lunch	Snack	Dinner	Snack	Bedtime	Night	Notes
Blood Sugar									
Insulin Dose									
Grams Carb									
Activity									

Date:	Breakfast	Snack	Lunch	Snack	Dinner	Snack	Bedtime	Night	Notes
Blood Sugar									
Insulin Dose									
Grams Carb									
Activity									

Date:	Breakfast	Snack	Lunch	Snack	Dinner	Snack	Bedtime	Night	Notes
Blood Sugar									
Insulin Dose									
Grams Carb									
Activity									

Date:	Breakfast	Snack	Lunch	Snack	Dinner	Snack	Bedtime	Night	Notes
Blood Sugar									
Insulin Dose									
Grams Carb									
Activity									

Date:	Breakfast	Snack	Lunch	Snack	Dinner	Snack	Bedtime	Night	Notes
Blood Sugar									
Insulin Dose									
Grams Carb									
Activity									

Weekly Diabetes Record

Name: _____

Date:	Breakfast	Snack	Lunch	Snack	Dinner	Snack	Bedtime	Night	Notes
Blood Sugar									
Insulin Dose									
Grams Carb									
Activity									

Date:	Breakfast	Snack	Lunch	Snack	Dinner	Snack	Bedtime	Night	Notes
Blood Sugar									
Insulin Dose									
Grams Carb									
Activity									

Date:	Breakfast	Snack	Lunch	Snack	Dinner	Snack	Bedtime	Night	Notes
Blood Sugar									
Insulin Dose									
Grams Carb									
Activity									

Date:	Breakfast	Snack	Lunch	Snack	Dinner	Snack	Bedtime	Night	Notes
Blood Sugar									
Insulin Dose									
Grams Carb									
Activity									

Date:	Breakfast	Snack	Lunch	Snack	Dinner	Snack	Bedtime	Night	Notes
Blood Sugar									
Insulin Dose									
Grams Carb									
Activity									

Date:	Breakfast	Snack	Lunch	Snack	Dinner	Snack	Bedtime	Night	Notes
Blood Sugar									
Insulin Dose									
Grams Carb									
Activity									

Date:	Breakfast	Snack	Lunch	Snack	Dinner	Snack	Bedtime	Night	Notes
Blood Sugar									
Insulin Dose									
Grams Carb									
Activity									

Weekly Diabetes Record

Name:

Date:	Breakfast	Snack	Lunch	Snack	Dinner	Snack	Bedtime	Night	Notes
Blood Sugar									
Insulin Dose									
Grams Carb									
Activity									

Date:	Breakfast	Snack	Lunch	Snack	Dinner	Snack	Bedtime	Night	Notes
Blood Sugar									
Insulin Dose									
Grams Carb									
Activity									

Date:	Breakfast	Snack	Lunch	Snack	Dinner	Snack	Bedtime	Night	Notes
Blood Sugar									
Insulin Dose									
Grams Carb									
Activity									

Date:	Breakfast	Snack	Lunch	Snack	Dinner	Snack	Bedtime	Night	Notes
Blood Sugar									
Insulin Dose									
Grams Carb									
Activity									

Date:	Breakfast	Snack	Lunch	Snack	Dinner	Snack	Bedtime	Night	Notes
Blood Sugar									
Insulin Dose									
Grams Carb									
Activity									

Date:	Breakfast	Snack	Lunch	Snack	Dinner	Snack	Bedtime	Night	Notes
Blood Sugar									
Insulin Dose									
Grams Carb									
Activity									

Date:	Breakfast	Snack	Lunch	Snack	Dinner	Snack	Bedtime	Night	Notes
Blood Sugar									
Insulin Dose									
Grams Carb									
Activity									

Weekly Diabetes Record

Name: _____

Date:	Breakfast	Snack	Lunch	Snack	Dinner	Snack	Bedtime	Night	Notes
Blood Sugar									
Insulin Dose									
Grams Carb									
Activity									

Date:	Breakfast	Snack	Lunch	Snack	Dinner	Snack	Bedtime	Night	Notes
Blood Sugar									
Insulin Dose									
Grams Carb									
Activity									

Date:	Breakfast	Snack	Lunch	Snack	Dinner	Snack	Bedtime	Night	Notes
Blood Sugar									
Insulin Dose									
Grams Carb									
Activity									

Date:	Breakfast	Snack	Lunch	Snack	Dinner	Snack	Bedtime	Night	Notes
Blood Sugar									
Insulin Dose									
Grams Carb									
Activity									

Date:	Breakfast	Snack	Lunch	Snack	Dinner	Snack	Bedtime	Night	Notes
Blood Sugar									
Insulin Dose									
Grams Carb									
Activity									

Date:	Breakfast	Snack	Lunch	Snack	Dinner	Snack	Bedtime	Night	Notes
Blood Sugar									
Insulin Dose									
Grams Carb									
Activity									

Date:	Breakfast	Snack	Lunch	Snack	Dinner	Snack	Bedtime	Night	Notes
Blood Sugar									
Insulin Dose									
Grams Carb									
Activity									

Weekly Diabetes Record

Name:

Date:	Breakfast	Snack	Lunch	Snack	Dinner	Snack	Bedtime	Night	Notes
Blood Sugar									
Insulin Dose									
Grams Carb									
Activity									

Date:	Breakfast	Snack	Lunch	Snack	Dinner	Snack	Bedtime	Night	Notes
Blood Sugar									
Insulin Dose									
Grams Carb									
Activity									

Date:	Breakfast	Snack	Lunch	Snack	Dinner	Snack	Bedtime	Night	Notes
Blood Sugar									
Insulin Dose									
Grams Carb									
Activity									

Date:	Breakfast	Snack	Lunch	Snack	Dinner	Snack	Bedtime	Night	Notes
Blood Sugar									
Insulin Dose									
Grams Carb									
Activity									

Date:	Breakfast	Snack	Lunch	Snack	Dinner	Snack	Bedtime	Night	Notes
Blood Sugar									
Insulin Dose									
Grams Carb									
Activity									

Date:	Breakfast	Snack	Lunch	Snack	Dinner	Snack	Bedtime	Night	Notes
Blood Sugar									
Insulin Dose									
Grams Carb									
Activity									

Date:	Breakfast	Snack	Lunch	Snack	Dinner	Snack	Bedtime	Night	Notes
Blood Sugar									
Insulin Dose									
Grams Carb									
Activity									

Weekly Diabetes Record

Name: _____

Date:	Breakfast	Snack	Lunch	Snack	Dinner	Snack	Bedtime	Night	Notes
Blood Sugar									
Insulin Dose									
Grams Carb									
Activity									

Date:	Breakfast	Snack	Lunch	Snack	Dinner	Snack	Bedtime	Night	Notes
Blood Sugar									
Insulin Dose									
Grams Carb									
Activity									

Date:	Breakfast	Snack	Lunch	Snack	Dinner	Snack	Bedtime	Night	Notes
Blood Sugar									
Insulin Dose									
Grams Carb									
Activity									

Date:	Breakfast	Snack	Lunch	Snack	Dinner	Snack	Bedtime	Night	Notes
Blood Sugar									
Insulin Dose									
Grams Carb									
Activity									

Date:	Breakfast	Snack	Lunch	Snack	Dinner	Snack	Bedtime	Night	Notes
Blood Sugar									
Insulin Dose									
Grams Carb									
Activity									

Date:	Breakfast	Snack	Lunch	Snack	Dinner	Snack	Bedtime	Night	Notes
Blood Sugar									
Insulin Dose									
Grams Carb									
Activity									

Date:	Breakfast	Snack	Lunch	Snack	Dinner	Snack	Bedtime	Night	Notes
Blood Sugar									
Insulin Dose									
Grams Carb									
Activity									

Weekly Diabetes Record

Name:

Date:	Breakfast	Snack	Lunch	Snack	Dinner	Snack	Bedtime	Night	Notes
Blood Sugar									
Insulin Dose									
Grams Carb									
Activity									

Date:	Breakfast	Snack	Lunch	Snack	Dinner	Snack	Bedtime	Night	Notes
Blood Sugar									
Insulin Dose									
Grams Carb									
Activity									

Date:	Breakfast	Snack	Lunch	Snack	Dinner	Snack	Bedtime	Night	Notes
Blood Sugar									
Insulin Dose									
Grams Carb									
Activity									

Date:	Breakfast	Snack	Lunch	Snack	Dinner	Snack	Bedtime	Night	Notes
Blood Sugar									
Insulin Dose									
Grams Carb									
Activity									

Date:	Breakfast	Snack	Lunch	Snack	Dinner	Snack	Bedtime	Night	Notes
Blood Sugar									
Insulin Dose									
Grams Carb									
Activity									

Date:	Breakfast	Snack	Lunch	Snack	Dinner	Snack	Bedtime	Night	Notes
Blood Sugar									
Insulin Dose									
Grams Carb									
Activity									

Date:	Breakfast	Snack	Lunch	Snack	Dinner	Snack	Bedtime	Night	Notes
Blood Sugar									
Insulin Dose									
Grams Carb									
Activity									

Weekly Diabetes Record

Name:

Date:	Breakfast	Snack	Lunch	Snack	Dinner	Snack	Bedtime	Night	Notes
Blood Sugar									
Insulin Dose									
Grams Carb									
Activity									

Date:	Breakfast	Snack	Lunch	Snack	Dinner	Snack	Bedtime	Night	Notes
Blood Sugar									
Insulin Dose									
Grams Carb									
Activity									

Date:	Breakfast	Snack	Lunch	Snack	Dinner	Snack	Bedtime	Night	Notes
Blood Sugar									
Insulin Dose									
Grams Carb									
Activity									

Date:	Breakfast	Snack	Lunch	Snack	Dinner	Snack	Bedtime	Night	Notes
Blood Sugar									
Insulin Dose									
Grams Carb									
Activity									

Date:	Breakfast	Snack	Lunch	Snack	Dinner	Snack	Bedtime	Night	Notes
Blood Sugar									
Insulin Dose									
Grams Carb									
Activity									

Date:	Breakfast	Snack	Lunch	Snack	Dinner	Snack	Bedtime	Night	Notes
Blood Sugar									
Insulin Dose									
Grams Carb									
Activity									

Date:	Breakfast	Snack	Lunch	Snack	Dinner	Snack	Bedtime	Night	Notes
Blood Sugar									
Insulin Dose									
Grams Carb									
Activity									

Weekly Diabetes Record

Name:

Date:	Breakfast	Snack	Lunch	Snack	Dinner	Snack	Bedtime	Night	Notes
Blood Sugar									
Insulin Dose									
Grams Carb									
Activity									

Date:	Breakfast	Snack	Lunch	Snack	Dinner	Snack	Bedtime	Night	Notes
Blood Sugar									
Insulin Dose									
Grams Carb									
Activity									

Date:	Breakfast	Snack	Lunch	Snack	Dinner	Snack	Bedtime	Night	Notes
Blood Sugar									
Insulin Dose									
Grams Carb									
Activity									

Date:	Breakfast	Snack	Lunch	Snack	Dinner	Snack	Bedtime	Night	Notes
Blood Sugar									
Insulin Dose									
Grams Carb									
Activity									

Date:	Breakfast	Snack	Lunch	Snack	Dinner	Snack	Bedtime	Night	Notes
Blood Sugar									
Insulin Dose									
Grams Carb									
Activity									

Date:	Breakfast	Snack	Lunch	Snack	Dinner	Snack	Bedtime	Night	Notes
Blood Sugar									
Insulin Dose									
Grams Carb									
Activity									

Date:	Breakfast	Snack	Lunch	Snack	Dinner	Snack	Bedtime	Night	Notes
Blood Sugar									
Insulin Dose									
Grams Carb									
Activity									

Weekly Diabetes Record

Name: _____

Date:	Breakfast	Snack	Lunch	Snack	Dinner	Snack	Bedtime	Night	Notes
Blood Sugar									
Insulin Dose									
Grams Carb									
Activity									

Date:	Breakfast	Snack	Lunch	Snack	Dinner	Snack	Bedtime	Night	Notes
Blood Sugar									
Insulin Dose									
Grams Carb									
Activity									

Date:	Breakfast	Snack	Lunch	Snack	Dinner	Snack	Bedtime	Night	Notes
Blood Sugar									
Insulin Dose									
Grams Carb									
Activity									

Date:	Breakfast	Snack	Lunch	Snack	Dinner	Snack	Bedtime	Night	Notes
Blood Sugar									
Insulin Dose									
Grams Carb									
Activity									

Date:	Breakfast	Snack	Lunch	Snack	Dinner	Snack	Bedtime	Night	Notes
Blood Sugar									
Insulin Dose									
Grams Carb									
Activity									

Date:	Breakfast	Snack	Lunch	Snack	Dinner	Snack	Bedtime	Night	Notes
Blood Sugar									
Insulin Dose									
Grams Carb									
Activity									

Date:	Breakfast	Snack	Lunch	Snack	Dinner	Snack	Bedtime	Night	Notes
Blood Sugar									
Insulin Dose									
Grams Carb									
Activity									

Weekly Diabetes Record

Name:

Date:	Breakfast	Snack	Lunch	Snack	Dinner	Snack	Bedtime	Night	Notes
Blood Sugar									
Insulin Dose									
Grams Carb									
Activity									

Date:	Breakfast	Snack	Lunch	Snack	Dinner	Snack	Bedtime	Night	Notes
Blood Sugar									
Insulin Dose									
Grams Carb									
Activity									

Date:	Breakfast	Snack	Lunch	Snack	Dinner	Snack	Bedtime	Night	Notes
Blood Sugar									
Insulin Dose									
Grams Carb									
Activity									

Date:	Breakfast	Snack	Lunch	Snack	Dinner	Snack	Bedtime	Night	Notes
Blood Sugar									
Insulin Dose									
Grams Carb									
Activity									

Date:	Breakfast	Snack	Lunch	Snack	Dinner	Snack	Bedtime	Night	Notes
Blood Sugar									
Insulin Dose									
Grams Carb									
Activity									

Date:	Breakfast	Snack	Lunch	Snack	Dinner	Snack	Bedtime	Night	Notes
Blood Sugar									
Insulin Dose									
Grams Carb									
Activity									

Date:	Breakfast	Snack	Lunch	Snack	Dinner	Snack	Bedtime	Night	Notes
Blood Sugar									
Insulin Dose									
Grams Carb									
Activity									

Weekly Diabetes Record

Name: _____

Date:	Breakfast	Snack	Lunch	Snack	Dinner	Snack	Bedtime	Night	Notes
Blood Sugar									
Insulin Dose									
Grams Carb									
Activity									

Date:	Breakfast	Snack	Lunch	Snack	Dinner	Snack	Bedtime	Night	Notes
Blood Sugar									
Insulin Dose									
Grams Carb									
Activity									

Date:	Breakfast	Snack	Lunch	Snack	Dinner	Snack	Bedtime	Night	Notes
Blood Sugar									
Insulin Dose									
Grams Carb									
Activity									

Date:	Breakfast	Snack	Lunch	Snack	Dinner	Snack	Bedtime	Night	Notes
Blood Sugar									
Insulin Dose									
Grams Carb									
Activity									

Date:	Breakfast	Snack	Lunch	Snack	Dinner	Snack	Bedtime	Night	Notes
Blood Sugar									
Insulin Dose									
Grams Carb									
Activity									

Date:	Breakfast	Snack	Lunch	Snack	Dinner	Snack	Bedtime	Night	Notes
Blood Sugar									
Insulin Dose									
Grams Carb									
Activity									

Date:	Breakfast	Snack	Lunch	Snack	Dinner	Snack	Bedtime	Night	Notes
Blood Sugar									
Insulin Dose									
Grams Carb									
Activity									

Weekly Diabetes Record

Name: _____

Date:	Breakfast	Snack	Lunch	Snack	Dinner	Snack	Bedtime	Night	Notes
Blood Sugar									
Insulin Dose									
Grams Carb									
Activity									

Date:	Breakfast	Snack	Lunch	Snack	Dinner	Snack	Bedtime	Night	Notes
Blood Sugar									
Insulin Dose									
Grams Carb									
Activity									

Date:	Breakfast	Snack	Lunch	Snack	Dinner	Snack	Bedtime	Night	Notes
Blood Sugar									
Insulin Dose									
Grams Carb									
Activity									

Date:	Breakfast	Snack	Lunch	Snack	Dinner	Snack	Bedtime	Night	Notes
Blood Sugar									
Insulin Dose									
Grams Carb									
Activity									

Date:	Breakfast	Snack	Lunch	Snack	Dinner	Snack	Bedtime	Night	Notes
Blood Sugar									
Insulin Dose									
Grams Carb									
Activity									

Date:	Breakfast	Snack	Lunch	Snack	Dinner	Snack	Bedtime	Night	Notes
Blood Sugar									
Insulin Dose									
Grams Carb									
Activity									

Date:	Breakfast	Snack	Lunch	Snack	Dinner	Snack	Bedtime	Night	Notes
Blood Sugar									
Insulin Dose									
Grams Carb									
Activity									

Weekly Diabetes Record

Name: _____

Date:	Breakfast	Snack	Lunch	Snack	Dinner	Snack	Bedtime	Night	Notes
Blood Sugar									
Insulin Dose									
Grams Carb									
Activity									

Date:	Breakfast	Snack	Lunch	Snack	Dinner	Snack	Bedtime	Night	Notes
Blood Sugar									
Insulin Dose									
Grams Carb									
Activity									

Date:	Breakfast	Snack	Lunch	Snack	Dinner	Snack	Bedtime	Night	Notes
Blood Sugar									
Insulin Dose									
Grams Carb									
Activity									

Date:	Breakfast	Snack	Lunch	Snack	Dinner	Snack	Bedtime	Night	Notes
Blood Sugar									
Insulin Dose									
Grams Carb									
Activity									

Date:	Breakfast	Snack	Lunch	Snack	Dinner	Snack	Bedtime	Night	Notes
Blood Sugar									
Insulin Dose									
Grams Carb									
Activity									

Date:	Breakfast	Snack	Lunch	Snack	Dinner	Snack	Bedtime	Night	Notes
Blood Sugar									
Insulin Dose									
Grams Carb									
Activity									

Date:	Breakfast	Snack	Lunch	Snack	Dinner	Snack	Bedtime	Night	Notes
Blood Sugar									
Insulin Dose									
Grams Carb									
Activity									

Weekly Diabetes Record

Name:

Date:	Breakfast	Snack	Lunch	Snack	Dinner	Snack	Bedtime	Night	Notes
Blood Sugar									
Insulin Dose									
Grams Carb									
Activity									

Date:	Breakfast	Snack	Lunch	Snack	Dinner	Snack	Bedtime	Night	Notes
Blood Sugar									
Insulin Dose									
Grams Carb									
Activity									

Date:	Breakfast	Snack	Lunch	Snack	Dinner	Snack	Bedtime	Night	Notes
Blood Sugar									
Insulin Dose									
Grams Carb									
Activity									

Date:	Breakfast	Snack	Lunch	Snack	Dinner	Snack	Bedtime	Night	Notes
Blood Sugar									
Insulin Dose									
Grams Carb									
Activity									

Date:	Breakfast	Snack	Lunch	Snack	Dinner	Snack	Bedtime	Night	Notes
Blood Sugar									
Insulin Dose									
Grams Carb									
Activity									

Date:	Breakfast	Snack	Lunch	Snack	Dinner	Snack	Bedtime	Night	Notes
Blood Sugar									
Insulin Dose									
Grams Carb									
Activity									

Date:	Breakfast	Snack	Lunch	Snack	Dinner	Snack	Bedtime	Night	Notes
Blood Sugar									
Insulin Dose									
Grams Carb									
Activity									

Weekly Diabetes Record

Name: _____

Date:	Breakfast	Snack	Lunch	Snack	Dinner	Snack	Bedtime	Night	Notes
Blood Sugar									
Insulin Dose									
Grams Carb									
Activity									

Date:	Breakfast	Snack	Lunch	Snack	Dinner	Snack	Bedtime	Night	Notes
Blood Sugar									
Insulin Dose									
Grams Carb									
Activity									

Date:	Breakfast	Snack	Lunch	Snack	Dinner	Snack	Bedtime	Night	Notes
Blood Sugar									
Insulin Dose									
Grams Carb									
Activity									

Date:	Breakfast	Snack	Lunch	Snack	Dinner	Snack	Bedtime	Night	Notes
Blood Sugar									
Insulin Dose									
Grams Carb									
Activity									

Date:	Breakfast	Snack	Lunch	Snack	Dinner	Snack	Bedtime	Night	Notes
Blood Sugar									
Insulin Dose									
Grams Carb									
Activity									

Date:	Breakfast	Snack	Lunch	Snack	Dinner	Snack	Bedtime	Night	Notes
Blood Sugar									
Insulin Dose									
Grams Carb									
Activity									

Date:	Breakfast	Snack	Lunch	Snack	Dinner	Snack	Bedtime	Night	Notes
Blood Sugar									
Insulin Dose									
Grams Carb									
Activity									

Weekly Diabetes Record

Name:

Date:	Breakfast	Snack	Lunch	Snack	Dinner	Snack	Bedtime	Night	Notes
Blood Sugar									
Insulin Dose									
Grams Carb									
Activity									

Date:	Breakfast	Snack	Lunch	Snack	Dinner	Snack	Bedtime	Night	Notes
Blood Sugar									
Insulin Dose									
Grams Carb									
Activity									

Date:	Breakfast	Snack	Lunch	Snack	Dinner	Snack	Bedtime	Night	Notes
Blood Sugar									
Insulin Dose									
Grams Carb									
Activity									

Date:	Breakfast	Snack	Lunch	Snack	Dinner	Snack	Bedtime	Night	Notes
Blood Sugar									
Insulin Dose									
Grams Carb									
Activity									

Date:	Breakfast	Snack	Lunch	Snack	Dinner	Snack	Bedtime	Night	Notes
Blood Sugar									
Insulin Dose									
Grams Carb									
Activity									

Date:	Breakfast	Snack	Lunch	Snack	Dinner	Snack	Bedtime	Night	Notes
Blood Sugar									
Insulin Dose									
Grams Carb									
Activity									

Date:	Breakfast	Snack	Lunch	Snack	Dinner	Snack	Bedtime	Night	Notes
Blood Sugar									
Insulin Dose									
Grams Carb									
Activity									

Weekly Diabetes Record

Name: _____

Date:	Breakfast	Snack	Lunch	Snack	Dinner	Snack	Bedtime	Night	Notes
Blood Sugar									
Insulin Dose									
Grams Carb									
Activity									

Date:	Breakfast	Snack	Lunch	Snack	Dinner	Snack	Bedtime	Night	Notes
Blood Sugar									
Insulin Dose									
Grams Carb									
Activity									

Date:	Breakfast	Snack	Lunch	Snack	Dinner	Snack	Bedtime	Night	Notes
Blood Sugar									
Insulin Dose									
Grams Carb									
Activity									

Date:	Breakfast	Snack	Lunch	Snack	Dinner	Snack	Bedtime	Night	Notes
Blood Sugar									
Insulin Dose									
Grams Carb									
Activity									

Date:	Breakfast	Snack	Lunch	Snack	Dinner	Snack	Bedtime	Night	Notes
Blood Sugar									
Insulin Dose									
Grams Carb									
Activity									

Date:	Breakfast	Snack	Lunch	Snack	Dinner	Snack	Bedtime	Night	Notes
Blood Sugar									
Insulin Dose									
Grams Carb									
Activity									

Date:	Breakfast	Snack	Lunch	Snack	Dinner	Snack	Bedtime	Night	Notes
Blood Sugar									
Insulin Dose									
Grams Carb									
Activity									

Weekly Diabetes Record

Name:

Date:	Breakfast	Snack	Lunch	Snack	Dinner	Snack	Bedtime	Night	Notes
Blood Sugar									
Insulin Dose									
Grams Carb									
Activity									

Date:	Breakfast	Snack	Lunch	Snack	Dinner	Snack	Bedtime	Night	Notes
Blood Sugar									
Insulin Dose									
Grams Carb									
Activity									

Date:	Breakfast	Snack	Lunch	Snack	Dinner	Snack	Bedtime	Night	Notes
Blood Sugar									
Insulin Dose									
Grams Carb									
Activity									

Date:	Breakfast	Snack	Lunch	Snack	Dinner	Snack	Bedtime	Night	Notes
Blood Sugar									
Insulin Dose									
Grams Carb									
Activity									

Date:	Breakfast	Snack	Lunch	Snack	Dinner	Snack	Bedtime	Night	Notes
Blood Sugar									
Insulin Dose									
Grams Carb									
Activity									

Date:	Breakfast	Snack	Lunch	Snack	Dinner	Snack	Bedtime	Night	Notes
Blood Sugar									
Insulin Dose									
Grams Carb									
Activity									

Date:	Breakfast	Snack	Lunch	Snack	Dinner	Snack	Bedtime	Night	Notes
Blood Sugar									
Insulin Dose									
Grams Carb									
Activity									

Weekly Diabetes Record

Name: _____

Date:	Breakfast	Snack	Lunch	Snack	Dinner	Snack	Bedtime	Night	Notes
Blood Sugar									
Insulin Dose									
Grams Carb									
Activity									

Date:	Breakfast	Snack	Lunch	Snack	Dinner	Snack	Bedtime	Night	Notes
Blood Sugar									
Insulin Dose									
Grams Carb									
Activity									

Date:	Breakfast	Snack	Lunch	Snack	Dinner	Snack	Bedtime	Night	Notes
Blood Sugar									
Insulin Dose									
Grams Carb									
Activity									

Date:	Breakfast	Snack	Lunch	Snack	Dinner	Snack	Bedtime	Night	Notes
Blood Sugar									
Insulin Dose									
Grams Carb									
Activity									

Date:	Breakfast	Snack	Lunch	Snack	Dinner	Snack	Bedtime	Night	Notes
Blood Sugar									
Insulin Dose									
Grams Carb									
Activity									

Date:	Breakfast	Snack	Lunch	Snack	Dinner	Snack	Bedtime	Night	Notes
Blood Sugar									
Insulin Dose									
Grams Carb									
Activity									

Date:	Breakfast	Snack	Lunch	Snack	Dinner	Snack	Bedtime	Night	Notes
Blood Sugar									
Insulin Dose									
Grams Carb									
Activity									

Weekly Diabetes Record

Name: _____

Date:	Breakfast	Snack	Lunch	Snack	Dinner	Snack	Bedtime	Night	Notes
Blood Sugar									
Insulin Dose									
Grams Carb									
Activity									

Date:	Breakfast	Snack	Lunch	Snack	Dinner	Snack	Bedtime	Night	Notes
Blood Sugar									
Insulin Dose									
Grams Carb									
Activity									

Date:	Breakfast	Snack	Lunch	Snack	Dinner	Snack	Bedtime	Night	Notes
Blood Sugar									
Insulin Dose									
Grams Carb									
Activity									

Date:	Breakfast	Snack	Lunch	Snack	Dinner	Snack	Bedtime	Night	Notes
Blood Sugar									
Insulin Dose									
Grams Carb									
Activity									

Date:	Breakfast	Snack	Lunch	Snack	Dinner	Snack	Bedtime	Night	Notes
Blood Sugar									
Insulin Dose									
Grams Carb									
Activity									

Date:	Breakfast	Snack	Lunch	Snack	Dinner	Snack	Bedtime	Night	Notes
Blood Sugar									
Insulin Dose									
Grams Carb									
Activity									

Date:	Breakfast	Snack	Lunch	Snack	Dinner	Snack	Bedtime	Night	Notes
Blood Sugar									
Insulin Dose									
Grams Carb									
Activity									

Weekly Diabetes Record

Name: _____

Date:	Breakfast	Snack	Lunch	Snack	Dinner	Snack	Bedtime	Night	Notes
Blood Sugar									
Insulin Dose									
Grams Carb									
Activity									

Date:	Breakfast	Snack	Lunch	Snack	Dinner	Snack	Bedtime	Night	Notes
Blood Sugar									
Insulin Dose									
Grams Carb									
Activity									

Date:	Breakfast	Snack	Lunch	Snack	Dinner	Snack	Bedtime	Night	Notes
Blood Sugar									
Insulin Dose									
Grams Carb									
Activity									

Date:	Breakfast	Snack	Lunch	Snack	Dinner	Snack	Bedtime	Night	Notes
Blood Sugar									
Insulin Dose									
Grams Carb									
Activity									

Date:	Breakfast	Snack	Lunch	Snack	Dinner	Snack	Bedtime	Night	Notes
Blood Sugar									
Insulin Dose									
Grams Carb									
Activity									

Date:	Breakfast	Snack	Lunch	Snack	Dinner	Snack	Bedtime	Night	Notes
Blood Sugar									
Insulin Dose									
Grams Carb									
Activity									

Date:	Breakfast	Snack	Lunch	Snack	Dinner	Snack	Bedtime	Night	Notes
Blood Sugar									
Insulin Dose									
Grams Carb									
Activity									

Weekly Diabetes Record

Name:

Date:	Breakfast	Snack	Lunch	Snack	Dinner	Snack	Bedtime	Night	Notes
Blood Sugar									
Insulin Dose									
Grams Carb									
Activity									

Date:	Breakfast	Snack	Lunch	Snack	Dinner	Snack	Bedtime	Night	Notes
Blood Sugar									
Insulin Dose									
Grams Carb									
Activity									

Date:	Breakfast	Snack	Lunch	Snack	Dinner	Snack	Bedtime	Night	Notes
Blood Sugar									
Insulin Dose									
Grams Carb									
Activity									

Date:	Breakfast	Snack	Lunch	Snack	Dinner	Snack	Bedtime	Night	Notes
Blood Sugar									
Insulin Dose									
Grams Carb									
Activity									

Date:	Breakfast	Snack	Lunch	Snack	Dinner	Snack	Bedtime	Night	Notes
Blood Sugar									
Insulin Dose									
Grams Carb									
Activity									

Date:	Breakfast	Snack	Lunch	Snack	Dinner	Snack	Bedtime	Night	Notes
Blood Sugar									
Insulin Dose									
Grams Carb									
Activity									

Date:	Breakfast	Snack	Lunch	Snack	Dinner	Snack	Bedtime	Night	Notes
Blood Sugar									
Insulin Dose									
Grams Carb									
Activity									

Weekly Diabetes Record

Name: _____

Date:	Breakfast	Snack	Lunch	Snack	Dinner	Snack	Bedtime	Night	Notes
Blood Sugar									
Insulin Dose									
Grams Carb									
Activity									

Date:	Breakfast	Snack	Lunch	Snack	Dinner	Snack	Bedtime	Night	Notes
Blood Sugar									
Insulin Dose									
Grams Carb									
Activity									

Date:	Breakfast	Snack	Lunch	Snack	Dinner	Snack	Bedtime	Night	Notes
Blood Sugar									
Insulin Dose									
Grams Carb									
Activity									

Date:	Breakfast	Snack	Lunch	Snack	Dinner	Snack	Bedtime	Night	Notes
Blood Sugar									
Insulin Dose									
Grams Carb									
Activity									

Date:	Breakfast	Snack	Lunch	Snack	Dinner	Snack	Bedtime	Night	Notes
Blood Sugar									
Insulin Dose									
Grams Carb									
Activity									

Date:	Breakfast	Snack	Lunch	Snack	Dinner	Snack	Bedtime	Night	Notes
Blood Sugar									
Insulin Dose									
Grams Carb									
Activity									

Date:	Breakfast	Snack	Lunch	Snack	Dinner	Snack	Bedtime	Night	Notes
Blood Sugar									
Insulin Dose									
Grams Carb									
Activity									

Weekly Diabetes Record

Name:

Date:	Breakfast	Snack	Lunch	Snack	Dinner	Snack	Bedtime	Night	Notes
Blood Sugar									
Insulin Dose									
Grams Carb									
Activity									

Date:	Breakfast	Snack	Lunch	Snack	Dinner	Snack	Bedtime	Night	Notes
Blood Sugar									
Insulin Dose									
Grams Carb									
Activity									

Date:	Breakfast	Snack	Lunch	Snack	Dinner	Snack	Bedtime	Night	Notes
Blood Sugar									
Insulin Dose									
Grams Carb									
Activity									

Date:	Breakfast	Snack	Lunch	Snack	Dinner	Snack	Bedtime	Night	Notes
Blood Sugar									
Insulin Dose									
Grams Carb									
Activity									

Date:	Breakfast	Snack	Lunch	Snack	Dinner	Snack	Bedtime	Night	Notes
Blood Sugar									
Insulin Dose									
Grams Carb									
Activity									

Date:	Breakfast	Snack	Lunch	Snack	Dinner	Snack	Bedtime	Night	Notes
Blood Sugar									
Insulin Dose									
Grams Carb									
Activity									

Date:	Breakfast	Snack	Lunch	Snack	Dinner	Snack	Bedtime	Night	Notes
Blood Sugar									
Insulin Dose									
Grams Carb									
Activity									

Weekly Diabetes Record

Name:

Date:	Breakfast	Snack	Lunch	Snack	Dinner	Snack	Bedtime	Night	Notes
Blood Sugar									
Insulin Dose									
Grams Carb									
Activity									

Date:	Breakfast	Snack	Lunch	Snack	Dinner	Snack	Bedtime	Night	Notes
Blood Sugar									
Insulin Dose									
Grams Carb									
Activity									

Date:	Breakfast	Snack	Lunch	Snack	Dinner	Snack	Bedtime	Night	Notes
Blood Sugar									
Insulin Dose									
Grams Carb									
Activity									

Date:	Breakfast	Snack	Lunch	Snack	Dinner	Snack	Bedtime	Night	Notes
Blood Sugar									
Insulin Dose									
Grams Carb									
Activity									

Date:	Breakfast	Snack	Lunch	Snack	Dinner	Snack	Bedtime	Night	Notes
Blood Sugar									
Insulin Dose									
Grams Carb									
Activity									

Date:	Breakfast	Snack	Lunch	Snack	Dinner	Snack	Bedtime	Night	Notes
Blood Sugar									
Insulin Dose									
Grams Carb									
Activity									

Date:	Breakfast	Snack	Lunch	Snack	Dinner	Snack	Bedtime	Night	Notes
Blood Sugar									
Insulin Dose									
Grams Carb									
Activity									

Weekly Diabetes Record

Name: _____

Date:	Breakfast	Snack	Lunch	Snack	Dinner	Snack	Bedtime	Night	Notes
Blood Sugar									
Insulin Dose									
Grams Carb									
Activity									

Date:	Breakfast	Snack	Lunch	Snack	Dinner	Snack	Bedtime	Night	Notes
Blood Sugar									
Insulin Dose									
Grams Carb									
Activity									

Date:	Breakfast	Snack	Lunch	Snack	Dinner	Snack	Bedtime	Night	Notes
Blood Sugar									
Insulin Dose									
Grams Carb									
Activity									

Date:	Breakfast	Snack	Lunch	Snack	Dinner	Snack	Bedtime	Night	Notes
Blood Sugar									
Insulin Dose									
Grams Carb									
Activity									

Date:	Breakfast	Snack	Lunch	Snack	Dinner	Snack	Bedtime	Night	Notes
Blood Sugar									
Insulin Dose									
Grams Carb									
Activity									

Date:	Breakfast	Snack	Lunch	Snack	Dinner	Snack	Bedtime	Night	Notes
Blood Sugar									
Insulin Dose									
Grams Carb									
Activity									

Date:	Breakfast	Snack	Lunch	Snack	Dinner	Snack	Bedtime	Night	Notes
Blood Sugar									
Insulin Dose									
Grams Carb									
Activity									

Weekly Diabetes Record

Name:

Date:	Breakfast	Snack	Lunch	Snack	Dinner	Snack	Bedtime	Night	Notes
Blood Sugar									
Insulin Dose									
Grams Carb									
Activity									

Date:	Breakfast	Snack	Lunch	Snack	Dinner	Snack	Bedtime	Night	Notes
Blood Sugar									
Insulin Dose									
Grams Carb									
Activity									

Date:	Breakfast	Snack	Lunch	Snack	Dinner	Snack	Bedtime	Night	Notes
Blood Sugar									
Insulin Dose									
Grams Carb									
Activity									

Date:	Breakfast	Snack	Lunch	Snack	Dinner	Snack	Bedtime	Night	Notes
Blood Sugar									
Insulin Dose									
Grams Carb									
Activity									

Date:	Breakfast	Snack	Lunch	Snack	Dinner	Snack	Bedtime	Night	Notes
Blood Sugar									
Insulin Dose									
Grams Carb									
Activity									

Date:	Breakfast	Snack	Lunch	Snack	Dinner	Snack	Bedtime	Night	Notes
Blood Sugar									
Insulin Dose									
Grams Carb									
Activity									

Date:	Breakfast	Snack	Lunch	Snack	Dinner	Snack	Bedtime	Night	Notes
Blood Sugar									
Insulin Dose									
Grams Carb									
Activity									

Weekly Diabetes Record

Name:

Date:	Breakfast	Snack	Lunch	Snack	Dinner	Snack	Bedtime	Night	Notes
Blood Sugar									
Insulin Dose									
Grams Carb									
Activity									

Date:	Breakfast	Snack	Lunch	Snack	Dinner	Snack	Bedtime	Night	Notes
Blood Sugar									
Insulin Dose									
Grams Carb									
Activity									

Date:	Breakfast	Snack	Lunch	Snack	Dinner	Snack	Bedtime	Night	Notes
Blood Sugar									
Insulin Dose									
Grams Carb									
Activity									

Date:	Breakfast	Snack	Lunch	Snack	Dinner	Snack	Bedtime	Night	Notes
Blood Sugar									
Insulin Dose									
Grams Carb									
Activity									

Date:	Breakfast	Snack	Lunch	Snack	Dinner	Snack	Bedtime	Night	Notes
Blood Sugar									
Insulin Dose									
Grams Carb									
Activity									

Date:	Breakfast	Snack	Lunch	Snack	Dinner	Snack	Bedtime	Night	Notes
Blood Sugar									
Insulin Dose									
Grams Carb									
Activity									

Date:	Breakfast	Snack	Lunch	Snack	Dinner	Snack	Bedtime	Night	Notes
Blood Sugar									
Insulin Dose									
Grams Carb									
Activity									

Weekly Diabetes Record

Name: _____

Date:	Breakfast	Snack	Lunch	Snack	Dinner	Snack	Bedtime	Night	Notes
Blood Sugar									
Insulin Dose									
Grams Carb									
Activity									

Date:	Breakfast	Snack	Lunch	Snack	Dinner	Snack	Bedtime	Night	Notes
Blood Sugar									
Insulin Dose									
Grams Carb									
Activity									

Date:	Breakfast	Snack	Lunch	Snack	Dinner	Snack	Bedtime	Night	Notes
Blood Sugar									
Insulin Dose									
Grams Carb									
Activity									

Date:	Breakfast	Snack	Lunch	Snack	Dinner	Snack	Bedtime	Night	Notes
Blood Sugar									
Insulin Dose									
Grams Carb									
Activity									

Date:	Breakfast	Snack	Lunch	Snack	Dinner	Snack	Bedtime	Night	Notes
Blood Sugar									
Insulin Dose									
Grams Carb									
Activity									

Date:	Breakfast	Snack	Lunch	Snack	Dinner	Snack	Bedtime	Night	Notes
Blood Sugar									
Insulin Dose									
Grams Carb									
Activity									

Date:	Breakfast	Snack	Lunch	Snack	Dinner	Snack	Bedtime	Night	Notes
Blood Sugar									
Insulin Dose									
Grams Carb									
Activity									

Weekly Diabetes Record

Name:

Date:	Breakfast	Snack	Lunch	Snack	Dinner	Snack	Bedtime	Night	Notes
Blood Sugar									
Insulin Dose									
Grams Carb									
Activity									

Date:	Breakfast	Snack	Lunch	Snack	Dinner	Snack	Bedtime	Night	Notes
Blood Sugar									
Insulin Dose									
Grams Carb									
Activity									

Date:	Breakfast	Snack	Lunch	Snack	Dinner	Snack	Bedtime	Night	Notes
Blood Sugar									
Insulin Dose									
Grams Carb									
Activity									

Date:	Breakfast	Snack	Lunch	Snack	Dinner	Snack	Bedtime	Night	Notes
Blood Sugar									
Insulin Dose									
Grams Carb									
Activity									

Date:	Breakfast	Snack	Lunch	Snack	Dinner	Snack	Bedtime	Night	Notes
Blood Sugar									
Insulin Dose									
Grams Carb									
Activity									

Date:	Breakfast	Snack	Lunch	Snack	Dinner	Snack	Bedtime	Night	Notes
Blood Sugar									
Insulin Dose									
Grams Carb									
Activity									

Date:	Breakfast	Snack	Lunch	Snack	Dinner	Snack	Bedtime	Night	Notes
Blood Sugar									
Insulin Dose									
Grams Carb									
Activity									

Weekly Diabetes Record

Name: _____

Date:	Breakfast	Snack	Lunch	Snack	Dinner	Snack	Bedtime	Night	Notes
Blood Sugar									
Insulin Dose									
Grams Carb									
Activity									

Date:	Breakfast	Snack	Lunch	Snack	Dinner	Snack	Bedtime	Night	Notes
Blood Sugar									
Insulin Dose									
Grams Carb									
Activity									

Date:	Breakfast	Snack	Lunch	Snack	Dinner	Snack	Bedtime	Night	Notes
Blood Sugar									
Insulin Dose									
Grams Carb									
Activity									

Date:	Breakfast	Snack	Lunch	Snack	Dinner	Snack	Bedtime	Night	Notes
Blood Sugar									
Insulin Dose									
Grams Carb									
Activity									

Date:	Breakfast	Snack	Lunch	Snack	Dinner	Snack	Bedtime	Night	Notes
Blood Sugar									
Insulin Dose									
Grams Carb									
Activity									

Date:	Breakfast	Snack	Lunch	Snack	Dinner	Snack	Bedtime	Night	Notes
Blood Sugar									
Insulin Dose									
Grams Carb									
Activity									

Date:	Breakfast	Snack	Lunch	Snack	Dinner	Snack	Bedtime	Night	Notes
Blood Sugar									
Insulin Dose									
Grams Carb									
Activity									

Weekly Diabetes Record

Name:

Date:	Breakfast	Snack	Lunch	Snack	Dinner	Snack	Bedtime	Night	Notes
Blood Sugar									
Insulin Dose									
Grams Carb									
Activity									

Date:	Breakfast	Snack	Lunch	Snack	Dinner	Snack	Bedtime	Night	Notes
Blood Sugar									
Insulin Dose									
Grams Carb									
Activity									

Date:	Breakfast	Snack	Lunch	Snack	Dinner	Snack	Bedtime	Night	Notes
Blood Sugar									
Insulin Dose									
Grams Carb									
Activity									

Date:	Breakfast	Snack	Lunch	Snack	Dinner	Snack	Bedtime	Night	Notes
Blood Sugar									
Insulin Dose									
Grams Carb									
Activity									

Date:	Breakfast	Snack	Lunch	Snack	Dinner	Snack	Bedtime	Night	Notes
Blood Sugar									
Insulin Dose									
Grams Carb									
Activity									

Date:	Breakfast	Snack	Lunch	Snack	Dinner	Snack	Bedtime	Night	Notes
Blood Sugar									
Insulin Dose									
Grams Carb									
Activity									

Date:	Breakfast	Snack	Lunch	Snack	Dinner	Snack	Bedtime	Night	Notes
Blood Sugar									
Insulin Dose									
Grams Carb									
Activity									

Weekly Diabetes Record

Name: _____

Date:	Breakfast	Snack	Lunch	Snack	Dinner	Snack	Bedtime	Night	Notes
Blood Sugar									
Insulin Dose									
Grams Carb									
Activity									

Date:	Breakfast	Snack	Lunch	Snack	Dinner	Snack	Bedtime	Night	Notes
Blood Sugar									
Insulin Dose									
Grams Carb									
Activity									

Date:	Breakfast	Snack	Lunch	Snack	Dinner	Snack	Bedtime	Night	Notes
Blood Sugar									
Insulin Dose									
Grams Carb									
Activity									

Date:	Breakfast	Snack	Lunch	Snack	Dinner	Snack	Bedtime	Night	Notes
Blood Sugar									
Insulin Dose									
Grams Carb									
Activity									

Date:	Breakfast	Snack	Lunch	Snack	Dinner	Snack	Bedtime	Night	Notes
Blood Sugar									
Insulin Dose									
Grams Carb									
Activity									

Date:	Breakfast	Snack	Lunch	Snack	Dinner	Snack	Bedtime	Night	Notes
Blood Sugar									
Insulin Dose									
Grams Carb									
Activity									

Date:	Breakfast	Snack	Lunch	Snack	Dinner	Snack	Bedtime	Night	Notes
Blood Sugar									
Insulin Dose									
Grams Carb									
Activity									

Weekly Diabetes Record

Name:

Date:	Breakfast	Snack	Lunch	Snack	Dinner	Snack	Bedtime	Night	Notes
Blood Sugar									
Insulin Dose									
Grams Carb									
Activity									

Date:	Breakfast	Snack	Lunch	Snack	Dinner	Snack	Bedtime	Night	Notes
Blood Sugar									
Insulin Dose									
Grams Carb									
Activity									

Date:	Breakfast	Snack	Lunch	Snack	Dinner	Snack	Bedtime	Night	Notes
Blood Sugar									
Insulin Dose									
Grams Carb									
Activity									

Date:	Breakfast	Snack	Lunch	Snack	Dinner	Snack	Bedtime	Night	Notes
Blood Sugar									
Insulin Dose									
Grams Carb									
Activity									

Date:	Breakfast	Snack	Lunch	Snack	Dinner	Snack	Bedtime	Night	Notes
Blood Sugar									
Insulin Dose									
Grams Carb									
Activity									

Date:	Breakfast	Snack	Lunch	Snack	Dinner	Snack	Bedtime	Night	Notes
Blood Sugar									
Insulin Dose									
Grams Carb									
Activity									

Date:	Breakfast	Snack	Lunch	Snack	Dinner	Snack	Bedtime	Night	Notes
Blood Sugar									
Insulin Dose									
Grams Carb									
Activity									

Weekly Diabetes Record

Name: _____

Date:	Breakfast	Snack	Lunch	Snack	Dinner	Snack	Bedtime	Night	Notes
Blood Sugar									
Insulin Dose									
Grams Carb									
Activity									

Date:	Breakfast	Snack	Lunch	Snack	Dinner	Snack	Bedtime	Night	Notes
Blood Sugar									
Insulin Dose									
Grams Carb									
Activity									

Date:	Breakfast	Snack	Lunch	Snack	Dinner	Snack	Bedtime	Night	Notes
Blood Sugar									
Insulin Dose									
Grams Carb									
Activity									

Date:	Breakfast	Snack	Lunch	Snack	Dinner	Snack	Bedtime	Night	Notes
Blood Sugar									
Insulin Dose									
Grams Carb									
Activity									

Date:	Breakfast	Snack	Lunch	Snack	Dinner	Snack	Bedtime	Night	Notes
Blood Sugar									
Insulin Dose									
Grams Carb									
Activity									

Date:	Breakfast	Snack	Lunch	Snack	Dinner	Snack	Bedtime	Night	Notes
Blood Sugar									
Insulin Dose									
Grams Carb									
Activity									

Date:	Breakfast	Snack	Lunch	Snack	Dinner	Snack	Bedtime	Night	Notes
Blood Sugar									
Insulin Dose									
Grams Carb									
Activity									

Weekly Diabetes Record

Name:

Date:	Breakfast	Snack	Lunch	Snack	Dinner	Snack	Bedtime	Night	Notes
Blood Sugar									
Insulin Dose									
Grams Carb									
Activity									

Date:	Breakfast	Snack	Lunch	Snack	Dinner	Snack	Bedtime	Night	Notes
Blood Sugar									
Insulin Dose									
Grams Carb									
Activity									

Date:	Breakfast	Snack	Lunch	Snack	Dinner	Snack	Bedtime	Night	Notes
Blood Sugar									
Insulin Dose									
Grams Carb									
Activity									

Date:	Breakfast	Snack	Lunch	Snack	Dinner	Snack	Bedtime	Night	Notes
Blood Sugar									
Insulin Dose									
Grams Carb									
Activity									

Date:	Breakfast	Snack	Lunch	Snack	Dinner	Snack	Bedtime	Night	Notes
Blood Sugar									
Insulin Dose									
Grams Carb									
Activity									

Date:	Breakfast	Snack	Lunch	Snack	Dinner	Snack	Bedtime	Night	Notes
Blood Sugar									
Insulin Dose									
Grams Carb									
Activity									

Date:	Breakfast	Snack	Lunch	Snack	Dinner	Snack	Bedtime	Night	Notes
Blood Sugar									
Insulin Dose									
Grams Carb									
Activity									

Weekly Diabetes Record

Name: _____

Date:	Breakfast	Snack	Lunch	Snack	Dinner	Snack	Bedtime	Night	Notes
Blood Sugar									
Insulin Dose									
Grams Carb									
Activity									

Date:	Breakfast	Snack	Lunch	Snack	Dinner	Snack	Bedtime	Night	Notes
Blood Sugar									
Insulin Dose									
Grams Carb									
Activity									

Date:	Breakfast	Snack	Lunch	Snack	Dinner	Snack	Bedtime	Night	Notes
Blood Sugar									
Insulin Dose									
Grams Carb									
Activity									

Date:	Breakfast	Snack	Lunch	Snack	Dinner	Snack	Bedtime	Night	Notes
Blood Sugar									
Insulin Dose									
Grams Carb									
Activity									

Date:	Breakfast	Snack	Lunch	Snack	Dinner	Snack	Bedtime	Night	Notes
Blood Sugar									
Insulin Dose									
Grams Carb									
Activity									

Date:	Breakfast	Snack	Lunch	Snack	Dinner	Snack	Bedtime	Night	Notes
Blood Sugar									
Insulin Dose									
Grams Carb									
Activity									

Date:	Breakfast	Snack	Lunch	Snack	Dinner	Snack	Bedtime	Night	Notes
Blood Sugar									
Insulin Dose									
Grams Carb									
Activity									

Weekly Diabetes Record

Name: _____

Date:	Breakfast	Snack	Lunch	Snack	Dinner	Snack	Bedtime	Night	Notes
Blood Sugar									
Insulin Dose									
Grams Carb									
Activity									

Date:	Breakfast	Snack	Lunch	Snack	Dinner	Snack	Bedtime	Night	Notes
Blood Sugar									
Insulin Dose									
Grams Carb									
Activity									

Date:	Breakfast	Snack	Lunch	Snack	Dinner	Snack	Bedtime	Night	Notes
Blood Sugar									
Insulin Dose									
Grams Carb									
Activity									

Date:	Breakfast	Snack	Lunch	Snack	Dinner	Snack	Bedtime	Night	Notes
Blood Sugar									
Insulin Dose									
Grams Carb									
Activity									

Date:	Breakfast	Snack	Lunch	Snack	Dinner	Snack	Bedtime	Night	Notes
Blood Sugar									
Insulin Dose									
Grams Carb									
Activity									

Date:	Breakfast	Snack	Lunch	Snack	Dinner	Snack	Bedtime	Night	Notes
Blood Sugar									
Insulin Dose									
Grams Carb									
Activity									

Date:	Breakfast	Snack	Lunch	Snack	Dinner	Snack	Bedtime	Night	Notes
Blood Sugar									
Insulin Dose									
Grams Carb									
Activity									

Weekly Diabetes Record

Name: _____

Date:	Breakfast	Snack	Lunch	Snack	Dinner	Snack	Bedtime	Night	Notes
Blood Sugar									
Insulin Dose									
Grams Carb									
Activity									

Date:	Breakfast	Snack	Lunch	Snack	Dinner	Snack	Bedtime	Night	Notes
Blood Sugar									
Insulin Dose									
Grams Carb									
Activity									

Date:	Breakfast	Snack	Lunch	Snack	Dinner	Snack	Bedtime	Night	Notes
Blood Sugar									
Insulin Dose									
Grams Carb									
Activity									

Date:	Breakfast	Snack	Lunch	Snack	Dinner	Snack	Bedtime	Night	Notes
Blood Sugar									
Insulin Dose									
Grams Carb									
Activity									

Date:	Breakfast	Snack	Lunch	Snack	Dinner	Snack	Bedtime	Night	Notes
Blood Sugar									
Insulin Dose									
Grams Carb									
Activity									

Date:	Breakfast	Snack	Lunch	Snack	Dinner	Snack	Bedtime	Night	Notes
Blood Sugar									
Insulin Dose									
Grams Carb									
Activity									

Date:	Breakfast	Snack	Lunch	Snack	Dinner	Snack	Bedtime	Night	Notes
Blood Sugar									
Insulin Dose									
Grams Carb									
Activity									

Weekly Diabetes Record

Name:

Date:	Breakfast	Snack	Lunch	Snack	Dinner	Snack	Bedtime	Night	Notes
Blood Sugar									
Insulin Dose									
Grams Carb									
Activity									

Date:	Breakfast	Snack	Lunch	Snack	Dinner	Snack	Bedtime	Night	Notes
Blood Sugar									
Insulin Dose									
Grams Carb									
Activity									

Date:	Breakfast	Snack	Lunch	Snack	Dinner	Snack	Bedtime	Night	Notes
Blood Sugar									
Insulin Dose									
Grams Carb									
Activity									

Date:	Breakfast	Snack	Lunch	Snack	Dinner	Snack	Bedtime	Night	Notes
Blood Sugar									
Insulin Dose									
Grams Carb									
Activity									

Date:	Breakfast	Snack	Lunch	Snack	Dinner	Snack	Bedtime	Night	Notes
Blood Sugar									
Insulin Dose									
Grams Carb									
Activity									

Date:	Breakfast	Snack	Lunch	Snack	Dinner	Snack	Bedtime	Night	Notes
Blood Sugar									
Insulin Dose									
Grams Carb									
Activity									

Date:	Breakfast	Snack	Lunch	Snack	Dinner	Snack	Bedtime	Night	Notes
Blood Sugar									
Insulin Dose									
Grams Carb									
Activity									

Weekly Diabetes Record

Name: _____

Date:	Breakfast	Snack	Lunch	Snack	Dinner	Snack	Bedtime	Night	Notes
Blood Sugar									
Insulin Dose									
Grams Carb									
Activity									

Date:	Breakfast	Snack	Lunch	Snack	Dinner	Snack	Bedtime	Night	Notes
Blood Sugar									
Insulin Dose									
Grams Carb									
Activity									

Date:	Breakfast	Snack	Lunch	Snack	Dinner	Snack	Bedtime	Night	Notes
Blood Sugar									
Insulin Dose									
Grams Carb									
Activity									

Date:	Breakfast	Snack	Lunch	Snack	Dinner	Snack	Bedtime	Night	Notes
Blood Sugar									
Insulin Dose									
Grams Carb									
Activity									

Date:	Breakfast	Snack	Lunch	Snack	Dinner	Snack	Bedtime	Night	Notes
Blood Sugar									
Insulin Dose									
Grams Carb									
Activity									

Date:	Breakfast	Snack	Lunch	Snack	Dinner	Snack	Bedtime	Night	Notes
Blood Sugar									
Insulin Dose									
Grams Carb									
Activity									

Date:	Breakfast	Snack	Lunch	Snack	Dinner	Snack	Bedtime	Night	Notes
Blood Sugar									
Insulin Dose									
Grams Carb									
Activity									

Weekly Diabetes Record

Name:

Date:	Breakfast	Snack	Lunch	Snack	Dinner	Snack	Bedtime	Night	Notes
Blood Sugar									
Insulin Dose									
Grams Carb									
Activity									

Date:	Breakfast	Snack	Lunch	Snack	Dinner	Snack	Bedtime	Night	Notes
Blood Sugar									
Insulin Dose									
Grams Carb									
Activity									

Date:	Breakfast	Snack	Lunch	Snack	Dinner	Snack	Bedtime	Night	Notes
Blood Sugar									
Insulin Dose									
Grams Carb									
Activity									

Date:	Breakfast	Snack	Lunch	Snack	Dinner	Snack	Bedtime	Night	Notes
Blood Sugar									
Insulin Dose									
Grams Carb									
Activity									

Date:	Breakfast	Snack	Lunch	Snack	Dinner	Snack	Bedtime	Night	Notes
Blood Sugar									
Insulin Dose									
Grams Carb									
Activity									

Date:	Breakfast	Snack	Lunch	Snack	Dinner	Snack	Bedtime	Night	Notes
Blood Sugar									
Insulin Dose									
Grams Carb									
Activity									

Date:	Breakfast	Snack	Lunch	Snack	Dinner	Snack	Bedtime	Night	Notes
Blood Sugar									
Insulin Dose									
Grams Carb									
Activity									

Weekly Diabetes Record

Name: _____

Date:	Breakfast	Snack	Lunch	Snack	Dinner	Snack	Bedtime	Night	Notes
Blood Sugar									
Insulin Dose									
Grams Carb									
Activity									

Date:	Breakfast	Snack	Lunch	Snack	Dinner	Snack	Bedtime	Night	Notes
Blood Sugar									
Insulin Dose									
Grams Carb									
Activity									

Date:	Breakfast	Snack	Lunch	Snack	Dinner	Snack	Bedtime	Night	Notes
Blood Sugar									
Insulin Dose									
Grams Carb									
Activity									

Date:	Breakfast	Snack	Lunch	Snack	Dinner	Snack	Bedtime	Night	Notes
Blood Sugar									
Insulin Dose									
Grams Carb									
Activity									

Date:	Breakfast	Snack	Lunch	Snack	Dinner	Snack	Bedtime	Night	Notes
Blood Sugar									
Insulin Dose									
Grams Carb									
Activity									

Date:	Breakfast	Snack	Lunch	Snack	Dinner	Snack	Bedtime	Night	Notes
Blood Sugar									
Insulin Dose									
Grams Carb									
Activity									

Date:	Breakfast	Snack	Lunch	Snack	Dinner	Snack	Bedtime	Night	Notes
Blood Sugar									
Insulin Dose									
Grams Carb									
Activity									

Weekly Diabetes Record

Name:

Date:	Breakfast	Snack	Lunch	Snack	Dinner	Snack	Bedtime	Night	Notes
Blood Sugar									
Insulin Dose									
Grams Carb									
Activity									

Date:	Breakfast	Snack	Lunch	Snack	Dinner	Snack	Bedtime	Night	Notes
Blood Sugar									
Insulin Dose									
Grams Carb									
Activity									

Date:	Breakfast	Snack	Lunch	Snack	Dinner	Snack	Bedtime	Night	Notes
Blood Sugar									
Insulin Dose									
Grams Carb									
Activity									

Date:	Breakfast	Snack	Lunch	Snack	Dinner	Snack	Bedtime	Night	Notes
Blood Sugar									
Insulin Dose									
Grams Carb									
Activity									

Date:	Breakfast	Snack	Lunch	Snack	Dinner	Snack	Bedtime	Night	Notes
Blood Sugar									
Insulin Dose									
Grams Carb									
Activity									

Date:	Breakfast	Snack	Lunch	Snack	Dinner	Snack	Bedtime	Night	Notes
Blood Sugar									
Insulin Dose									
Grams Carb									
Activity									

Date:	Breakfast	Snack	Lunch	Snack	Dinner	Snack	Bedtime	Night	Notes
Blood Sugar									
Insulin Dose									
Grams Carb									
Activity									

Weekly Diabetes Record

Name:

Date:	Breakfast	Snack	Lunch	Snack	Dinner	Snack	Bedtime	Night	Notes
Blood Sugar									
Insulin Dose									
Grams Carb									
Activity									

Date:	Breakfast	Snack	Lunch	Snack	Dinner	Snack	Bedtime	Night	Notes
Blood Sugar									
Insulin Dose									
Grams Carb									
Activity									

Date:	Breakfast	Snack	Lunch	Snack	Dinner	Snack	Bedtime	Night	Notes
Blood Sugar									
Insulin Dose									
Grams Carb									
Activity									

Date:	Breakfast	Snack	Lunch	Snack	Dinner	Snack	Bedtime	Night	Notes
Blood Sugar									
Insulin Dose									
Grams Carb									
Activity									

Date:	Breakfast	Snack	Lunch	Snack	Dinner	Snack	Bedtime	Night	Notes
Blood Sugar									
Insulin Dose									
Grams Carb									
Activity									

Date:	Breakfast	Snack	Lunch	Snack	Dinner	Snack	Bedtime	Night	Notes
Blood Sugar									
Insulin Dose									
Grams Carb									
Activity									

Date:	Breakfast	Snack	Lunch	Snack	Dinner	Snack	Bedtime	Night	Notes
Blood Sugar									
Insulin Dose									
Grams Carb									
Activity									

Weekly Diabetes Record

Name:

Date:	Breakfast	Snack	Lunch	Snack	Dinner	Snack	Bedtime	Night	Notes
Blood Sugar									
Insulin Dose									
Grams Carb									
Activity									

Date:	Breakfast	Snack	Lunch	Snack	Dinner	Snack	Bedtime	Night	Notes
Blood Sugar									
Insulin Dose									
Grams Carb									
Activity									

Date:	Breakfast	Snack	Lunch	Snack	Dinner	Snack	Bedtime	Night	Notes
Blood Sugar									
Insulin Dose									
Grams Carb									
Activity									

Date:	Breakfast	Snack	Lunch	Snack	Dinner	Snack	Bedtime	Night	Notes
Blood Sugar									
Insulin Dose									
Grams Carb									
Activity									

Date:	Breakfast	Snack	Lunch	Snack	Dinner	Snack	Bedtime	Night	Notes
Blood Sugar									
Insulin Dose									
Grams Carb									
Activity									

Date:	Breakfast	Snack	Lunch	Snack	Dinner	Snack	Bedtime	Night	Notes
Blood Sugar									
Insulin Dose									
Grams Carb									
Activity									

Date:	Breakfast	Snack	Lunch	Snack	Dinner	Snack	Bedtime	Night	Notes
Blood Sugar									
Insulin Dose									
Grams Carb									
Activity									

Weekly Diabetes Record

Name: _____

Date:	Breakfast	Snack	Lunch	Snack	Dinner	Snack	Bedtime	Night	Notes
Blood Sugar									
Insulin Dose									
Grams Carb									
Activity									

Date:	Breakfast	Snack	Lunch	Snack	Dinner	Snack	Bedtime	Night	Notes
Blood Sugar									
Insulin Dose									
Grams Carb									
Activity									

Date:	Breakfast	Snack	Lunch	Snack	Dinner	Snack	Bedtime	Night	Notes
Blood Sugar									
Insulin Dose									
Grams Carb									
Activity									

Date:	Breakfast	Snack	Lunch	Snack	Dinner	Snack	Bedtime	Night	Notes
Blood Sugar									
Insulin Dose									
Grams Carb									
Activity									

Date:	Breakfast	Snack	Lunch	Snack	Dinner	Snack	Bedtime	Night	Notes
Blood Sugar									
Insulin Dose									
Grams Carb									
Activity									

Date:	Breakfast	Snack	Lunch	Snack	Dinner	Snack	Bedtime	Night	Notes
Blood Sugar									
Insulin Dose									
Grams Carb									
Activity									

Date:	Breakfast	Snack	Lunch	Snack	Dinner	Snack	Bedtime	Night	Notes
Blood Sugar									
Insulin Dose									
Grams Carb									
Activity									

Weekly Diabetes Record

Name:

Date:	Breakfast	Snack	Lunch	Snack	Dinner	Snack	Bedtime	Night	Notes
Blood Sugar									
Insulin Dose									
Grams Carb									
Activity									

Date:	Breakfast	Snack	Lunch	Snack	Dinner	Snack	Bedtime	Night	Notes
Blood Sugar									
Insulin Dose									
Grams Carb									
Activity									

Date:	Breakfast	Snack	Lunch	Snack	Dinner	Snack	Bedtime	Night	Notes
Blood Sugar									
Insulin Dose									
Grams Carb									
Activity									

Date:	Breakfast	Snack	Lunch	Snack	Dinner	Snack	Bedtime	Night	Notes
Blood Sugar									
Insulin Dose									
Grams Carb									
Activity									

Date:	Breakfast	Snack	Lunch	Snack	Dinner	Snack	Bedtime	Night	Notes
Blood Sugar									
Insulin Dose									
Grams Carb									
Activity									

Date:	Breakfast	Snack	Lunch	Snack	Dinner	Snack	Bedtime	Night	Notes
Blood Sugar									
Insulin Dose									
Grams Carb									
Activity									

Date:	Breakfast	Snack	Lunch	Snack	Dinner	Snack	Bedtime	Night	Notes
Blood Sugar									
Insulin Dose									
Grams Carb									
Activity									

Weekly Diabetes Record

Name: _____

Date:	Breakfast	Snack	Lunch	Snack	Dinner	Snack	Bedtime	Night	Notes
Blood Sugar									
Insulin Dose									
Grams Carb									
Activity									

Date:	Breakfast	Snack	Lunch	Snack	Dinner	Snack	Bedtime	Night	Notes
Blood Sugar									
Insulin Dose									
Grams Carb									
Activity									

Date:	Breakfast	Snack	Lunch	Snack	Dinner	Snack	Bedtime	Night	Notes
Blood Sugar									
Insulin Dose									
Grams Carb									
Activity									

Date:	Breakfast	Snack	Lunch	Snack	Dinner	Snack	Bedtime	Night	Notes
Blood Sugar									
Insulin Dose									
Grams Carb									
Activity									

Date:	Breakfast	Snack	Lunch	Snack	Dinner	Snack	Bedtime	Night	Notes
Blood Sugar									
Insulin Dose									
Grams Carb									
Activity									

Date:	Breakfast	Snack	Lunch	Snack	Dinner	Snack	Bedtime	Night	Notes
Blood Sugar									
Insulin Dose									
Grams Carb									
Activity									

Date:	Breakfast	Snack	Lunch	Snack	Dinner	Snack	Bedtime	Night	Notes
Blood Sugar									
Insulin Dose									
Grams Carb									
Activity									

Weekly Diabetes Record

Name:

Date:	Breakfast	Snack	Lunch	Snack	Dinner	Snack	Bedtime	Night	Notes
Blood Sugar									
Insulin Dose									
Grams Carb									
Activity									

Date:	Breakfast	Snack	Lunch	Snack	Dinner	Snack	Bedtime	Night	Notes
Blood Sugar									
Insulin Dose									
Grams Carb									
Activity									

Date:	Breakfast	Snack	Lunch	Snack	Dinner	Snack	Bedtime	Night	Notes
Blood Sugar									
Insulin Dose									
Grams Carb									
Activity									

Date:	Breakfast	Snack	Lunch	Snack	Dinner	Snack	Bedtime	Night	Notes
Blood Sugar									
Insulin Dose									
Grams Carb									
Activity									

Date:	Breakfast	Snack	Lunch	Snack	Dinner	Snack	Bedtime	Night	Notes
Blood Sugar									
Insulin Dose									
Grams Carb									
Activity									

Date:	Breakfast	Snack	Lunch	Snack	Dinner	Snack	Bedtime	Night	Notes
Blood Sugar									
Insulin Dose									
Grams Carb									
Activity									

Date:	Breakfast	Snack	Lunch	Snack	Dinner	Snack	Bedtime	Night	Notes
Blood Sugar									
Insulin Dose									
Grams Carb									
Activity									

Weekly Diabetes Record

Name:

Date:	Breakfast	Snack	Lunch	Snack	Dinner	Snack	Bedtime	Night	Notes
Blood Sugar									
Insulin Dose									
Grams Carb									
Activity									

Date:	Breakfast	Snack	Lunch	Snack	Dinner	Snack	Bedtime	Night	Notes
Blood Sugar									
Insulin Dose									
Grams Carb									
Activity									

Date:	Breakfast	Snack	Lunch	Snack	Dinner	Snack	Bedtime	Night	Notes
Blood Sugar									
Insulin Dose									
Grams Carb									
Activity									

Date:	Breakfast	Snack	Lunch	Snack	Dinner	Snack	Bedtime	Night	Notes
Blood Sugar									
Insulin Dose									
Grams Carb									
Activity									

Date:	Breakfast	Snack	Lunch	Snack	Dinner	Snack	Bedtime	Night	Notes
Blood Sugar									
Insulin Dose									
Grams Carb									
Activity									

Date:	Breakfast	Snack	Lunch	Snack	Dinner	Snack	Bedtime	Night	Notes
Blood Sugar									
Insulin Dose									
Grams Carb									
Activity									

Date:	Breakfast	Snack	Lunch	Snack	Dinner	Snack	Bedtime	Night	Notes
Blood Sugar									
Insulin Dose									
Grams Carb									
Activity									

Weekly Diabetes Record

Name: _____

Date:	Breakfast	Snack	Lunch	Snack	Dinner	Snack	Bedtime	Night	Notes
Blood Sugar									
Insulin Dose									
Grams Carb									
Activity									

Date:	Breakfast	Snack	Lunch	Snack	Dinner	Snack	Bedtime	Night	Notes
Blood Sugar									
Insulin Dose									
Grams Carb									
Activity									

Date:	Breakfast	Snack	Lunch	Snack	Dinner	Snack	Bedtime	Night	Notes
Blood Sugar									
Insulin Dose									
Grams Carb									
Activity									

Date:	Breakfast	Snack	Lunch	Snack	Dinner	Snack	Bedtime	Night	Notes
Blood Sugar									
Insulin Dose									
Grams Carb									
Activity									

Date:	Breakfast	Snack	Lunch	Snack	Dinner	Snack	Bedtime	Night	Notes
Blood Sugar									
Insulin Dose									
Grams Carb									
Activity									

Date:	Breakfast	Snack	Lunch	Snack	Dinner	Snack	Bedtime	Night	Notes
Blood Sugar									
Insulin Dose									
Grams Carb									
Activity									

Date:	Breakfast	Snack	Lunch	Snack	Dinner	Snack	Bedtime	Night	Notes
Blood Sugar									
Insulin Dose									
Grams Carb									
Activity									

Weekly Diabetes Record

Name: _____

Date:	Breakfast	Snack	Lunch	Snack	Dinner	Snack	Bedtime	Night	Notes
Blood Sugar									
Insulin Dose									
Grams Carb									
Activity									

Date:	Breakfast	Snack	Lunch	Snack	Dinner	Snack	Bedtime	Night	Notes
Blood Sugar									
Insulin Dose									
Grams Carb									
Activity									

Date:	Breakfast	Snack	Lunch	Snack	Dinner	Snack	Bedtime	Night	Notes
Blood Sugar									
Insulin Dose									
Grams Carb									
Activity									

Date:	Breakfast	Snack	Lunch	Snack	Dinner	Snack	Bedtime	Night	Notes
Blood Sugar									
Insulin Dose									
Grams Carb									
Activity									

Date:	Breakfast	Snack	Lunch	Snack	Dinner	Snack	Bedtime	Night	Notes
Blood Sugar									
Insulin Dose									
Grams Carb									
Activity									

Date:	Breakfast	Snack	Lunch	Snack	Dinner	Snack	Bedtime	Night	Notes
Blood Sugar									
Insulin Dose									
Grams Carb									
Activity									

Date:	Breakfast	Snack	Lunch	Snack	Dinner	Snack	Bedtime	Night	Notes
Blood Sugar									
Insulin Dose									
Grams Carb									
Activity									

Weekly Diabetes Record

Name:

Date:	Breakfast	Snack	Lunch	Snack	Dinner	Snack	Bedtime	Night	Notes
Blood Sugar									
Insulin Dose									
Grams Carb									
Activity									

Date:	Breakfast	Snack	Lunch	Snack	Dinner	Snack	Bedtime	Night	Notes
Blood Sugar									
Insulin Dose									
Grams Carb									
Activity									

Date:	Breakfast	Snack	Lunch	Snack	Dinner	Snack	Bedtime	Night	Notes
Blood Sugar									
Insulin Dose									
Grams Carb									
Activity									

Date:	Breakfast	Snack	Lunch	Snack	Dinner	Snack	Bedtime	Night	Notes
Blood Sugar									
Insulin Dose									
Grams Carb									
Activity									

Date:	Breakfast	Snack	Lunch	Snack	Dinner	Snack	Bedtime	Night	Notes
Blood Sugar									
Insulin Dose									
Grams Carb									
Activity									

Date:	Breakfast	Snack	Lunch	Snack	Dinner	Snack	Bedtime	Night	Notes
Blood Sugar									
Insulin Dose									
Grams Carb									
Activity									

Date:	Breakfast	Snack	Lunch	Snack	Dinner	Snack	Bedtime	Night	Notes
Blood Sugar									
Insulin Dose									
Grams Carb									
Activity									

Weekly Diabetes Record

Name: _____

Date:	Breakfast	Snack	Lunch	Snack	Dinner	Snack	Bedtime	Night	Notes
Blood Sugar									
Insulin Dose									
Grams Carb									
Activity									

Date:	Breakfast	Snack	Lunch	Snack	Dinner	Snack	Bedtime	Night	Notes
Blood Sugar									
Insulin Dose									
Grams Carb									
Activity									

Date:	Breakfast	Snack	Lunch	Snack	Dinner	Snack	Bedtime	Night	Notes
Blood Sugar									
Insulin Dose									
Grams Carb									
Activity									

Date:	Breakfast	Snack	Lunch	Snack	Dinner	Snack	Bedtime	Night	Notes
Blood Sugar									
Insulin Dose									
Grams Carb									
Activity									

Date:	Breakfast	Snack	Lunch	Snack	Dinner	Snack	Bedtime	Night	Notes
Blood Sugar									
Insulin Dose									
Grams Carb									
Activity									

Date:	Breakfast	Snack	Lunch	Snack	Dinner	Snack	Bedtime	Night	Notes
Blood Sugar									
Insulin Dose									
Grams Carb									
Activity									

Date:	Breakfast	Snack	Lunch	Snack	Dinner	Snack	Bedtime	Night	Notes
Blood Sugar									
Insulin Dose									
Grams Carb									
Activity									

Weekly Diabetes Record

Name:

Date:	Breakfast	Snack	Lunch	Snack	Dinner	Snack	Bedtime	Night	Notes
Blood Sugar									
Insulin Dose									
Grams Carb									
Activity									

Date:	Breakfast	Snack	Lunch	Snack	Dinner	Snack	Bedtime	Night	Notes
Blood Sugar									
Insulin Dose									
Grams Carb									
Activity									

Date:	Breakfast	Snack	Lunch	Snack	Dinner	Snack	Bedtime	Night	Notes
Blood Sugar									
Insulin Dose									
Grams Carb									
Activity									

Date:	Breakfast	Snack	Lunch	Snack	Dinner	Snack	Bedtime	Night	Notes
Blood Sugar									
Insulin Dose									
Grams Carb									
Activity									

Date:	Breakfast	Snack	Lunch	Snack	Dinner	Snack	Bedtime	Night	Notes
Blood Sugar									
Insulin Dose									
Grams Carb									
Activity									

Date:	Breakfast	Snack	Lunch	Snack	Dinner	Snack	Bedtime	Night	Notes
Blood Sugar									
Insulin Dose									
Grams Carb									
Activity									

Date:	Breakfast	Snack	Lunch	Snack	Dinner	Snack	Bedtime	Night	Notes
Blood Sugar									
Insulin Dose									
Grams Carb									
Activity									

Weekly Diabetes Record

Name:

Date:	Breakfast	Snack	Lunch	Snack	Dinner	Snack	Bedtime	Night	Notes
Blood Sugar									
Insulin Dose									
Grams Carb									
Activity									

Date:	Breakfast	Snack	Lunch	Snack	Dinner	Snack	Bedtime	Night	Notes
Blood Sugar									
Insulin Dose									
Grams Carb									
Activity									

Date:	Breakfast	Snack	Lunch	Snack	Dinner	Snack	Bedtime	Night	Notes
Blood Sugar									
Insulin Dose									
Grams Carb									
Activity									

Date:	Breakfast	Snack	Lunch	Snack	Dinner	Snack	Bedtime	Night	Notes
Blood Sugar									
Insulin Dose									
Grams Carb									
Activity									

Date:	Breakfast	Snack	Lunch	Snack	Dinner	Snack	Bedtime	Night	Notes
Blood Sugar									
Insulin Dose									
Grams Carb									
Activity									

Date:	Breakfast	Snack	Lunch	Snack	Dinner	Snack	Bedtime	Night	Notes
Blood Sugar									
Insulin Dose									
Grams Carb									
Activity									

Date:	Breakfast	Snack	Lunch	Snack	Dinner	Snack	Bedtime	Night	Notes
Blood Sugar									
Insulin Dose									
Grams Carb									
Activity									

Weekly Diabetes Record

Name:

Date:	Breakfast	Snack	Lunch	Snack	Dinner	Snack	Bedtime	Night	Notes
Blood Sugar									
Insulin Dose									
Grams Carb									
Activity									

Date:	Breakfast	Snack	Lunch	Snack	Dinner	Snack	Bedtime	Night	Notes
Blood Sugar									
Insulin Dose									
Grams Carb									
Activity									

Date:	Breakfast	Snack	Lunch	Snack	Dinner	Snack	Bedtime	Night	Notes
Blood Sugar									
Insulin Dose									
Grams Carb									
Activity									

Date:	Breakfast	Snack	Lunch	Snack	Dinner	Snack	Bedtime	Night	Notes
Blood Sugar									
Insulin Dose									
Grams Carb									
Activity									

Date:	Breakfast	Snack	Lunch	Snack	Dinner	Snack	Bedtime	Night	Notes
Blood Sugar									
Insulin Dose									
Grams Carb									
Activity									

Date:	Breakfast	Snack	Lunch	Snack	Dinner	Snack	Bedtime	Night	Notes
Blood Sugar									
Insulin Dose									
Grams Carb									
Activity									

Date:	Breakfast	Snack	Lunch	Snack	Dinner	Snack	Bedtime	Night	Notes
Blood Sugar									
Insulin Dose									
Grams Carb									
Activity									

Weekly Diabetes Record

Name: _____

Date:	Breakfast	Snack	Lunch	Snack	Dinner	Snack	Bedtime	Night	Notes
Blood Sugar									
Insulin Dose									
Grams Carb									
Activity									

Date:	Breakfast	Snack	Lunch	Snack	Dinner	Snack	Bedtime	Night	Notes
Blood Sugar									
Insulin Dose									
Grams Carb									
Activity									

Date:	Breakfast	Snack	Lunch	Snack	Dinner	Snack	Bedtime	Night	Notes
Blood Sugar									
Insulin Dose									
Grams Carb									
Activity									

Date:	Breakfast	Snack	Lunch	Snack	Dinner	Snack	Bedtime	Night	Notes
Blood Sugar									
Insulin Dose									
Grams Carb									
Activity									

Date:	Breakfast	Snack	Lunch	Snack	Dinner	Snack	Bedtime	Night	Notes
Blood Sugar									
Insulin Dose									
Grams Carb									
Activity									

Date:	Breakfast	Snack	Lunch	Snack	Dinner	Snack	Bedtime	Night	Notes
Blood Sugar									
Insulin Dose									
Grams Carb									
Activity									

Date:	Breakfast	Snack	Lunch	Snack	Dinner	Snack	Bedtime	Night	Notes
Blood Sugar									
Insulin Dose									
Grams Carb									
Activity									

Weekly Diabetes Record

Name:

Date:	Breakfast	Snack	Lunch	Snack	Dinner	Snack	Bedtime	Night	Notes
Blood Sugar									
Insulin Dose									
Grams Carb									
Activity									

Date:	Breakfast	Snack	Lunch	Snack	Dinner	Snack	Bedtime	Night	Notes
Blood Sugar									
Insulin Dose									
Grams Carb									
Activity									

Date:	Breakfast	Snack	Lunch	Snack	Dinner	Snack	Bedtime	Night	Notes
Blood Sugar									
Insulin Dose									
Grams Carb									
Activity									

Date:	Breakfast	Snack	Lunch	Snack	Dinner	Snack	Bedtime	Night	Notes
Blood Sugar									
Insulin Dose									
Grams Carb									
Activity									

Date:	Breakfast	Snack	Lunch	Snack	Dinner	Snack	Bedtime	Night	Notes
Blood Sugar									
Insulin Dose									
Grams Carb									
Activity									

Date:	Breakfast	Snack	Lunch	Snack	Dinner	Snack	Bedtime	Night	Notes
Blood Sugar									
Insulin Dose									
Grams Carb									
Activity									

Date:	Breakfast	Snack	Lunch	Snack	Dinner	Snack	Bedtime	Night	Notes
Blood Sugar									
Insulin Dose									
Grams Carb									
Activity									

Weekly Diabetes Record

Name: _____

Date:	Breakfast	Snack	Lunch	Snack	Dinner	Snack	Bedtime	Night	Notes
Blood Sugar									
Insulin Dose									
Grams Carb									
Activity									

Date:	Breakfast	Snack	Lunch	Snack	Dinner	Snack	Bedtime	Night	Notes
Blood Sugar									
Insulin Dose									
Grams Carb									
Activity									

Date:	Breakfast	Snack	Lunch	Snack	Dinner	Snack	Bedtime	Night	Notes
Blood Sugar									
Insulin Dose									
Grams Carb									
Activity									

Date:	Breakfast	Snack	Lunch	Snack	Dinner	Snack	Bedtime	Night	Notes
Blood Sugar									
Insulin Dose									
Grams Carb									
Activity									

Date:	Breakfast	Snack	Lunch	Snack	Dinner	Snack	Bedtime	Night	Notes
Blood Sugar									
Insulin Dose									
Grams Carb									
Activity									

Date:	Breakfast	Snack	Lunch	Snack	Dinner	Snack	Bedtime	Night	Notes
Blood Sugar									
Insulin Dose									
Grams Carb									
Activity									

Date:	Breakfast	Snack	Lunch	Snack	Dinner	Snack	Bedtime	Night	Notes
Blood Sugar									
Insulin Dose									
Grams Carb									
Activity									

Weekly Diabetes Record

Name: _____

Date:	Breakfast	Snack	Lunch	Snack	Dinner	Snack	Bedtime	Night	Notes
Blood Sugar									
Insulin Dose									
Grams Carb									
Activity									

Date:	Breakfast	Snack	Lunch	Snack	Dinner	Snack	Bedtime	Night	Notes
Blood Sugar									
Insulin Dose									
Grams Carb									
Activity									

Date:	Breakfast	Snack	Lunch	Snack	Dinner	Snack	Bedtime	Night	Notes
Blood Sugar									
Insulin Dose									
Grams Carb									
Activity									

Date:	Breakfast	Snack	Lunch	Snack	Dinner	Snack	Bedtime	Night	Notes
Blood Sugar									
Insulin Dose									
Grams Carb									
Activity									

Date:	Breakfast	Snack	Lunch	Snack	Dinner	Snack	Bedtime	Night	Notes
Blood Sugar									
Insulin Dose									
Grams Carb									
Activity									

Date:	Breakfast	Snack	Lunch	Snack	Dinner	Snack	Bedtime	Night	Notes
Blood Sugar									
Insulin Dose									
Grams Carb									
Activity									

Date:	Breakfast	Snack	Lunch	Snack	Dinner	Snack	Bedtime	Night	Notes
Blood Sugar									
Insulin Dose									
Grams Carb									
Activity									

Printed in Great Britain
by Amazon

37784423R00066